Religions, Culture and Healthcare

Religions, Culture and Healthcare

A practical handbook for use in healthcare environments

Susan Hollins

Lead Chaplain
NHS National Chaplaincy Strategy

Foreword by
Surinder Sharma

National Director for Equality and Human Rights
Department of Health and the NHS

Radcliffe Publishing
Oxford • Seattle

Radcliffe Publishing Ltd
18 Marcham Road
Abingdon
Oxon OX14 1AA
United Kingdom

www.radcliffe-oxford.com
Electronic catalogue and worldwide online ordering facility.

62344986

British Library Cataloguing in Publication Data

A catalogue record for this book is available from the British Library.

ISBN-10 1 85775 755 6
ISBN-13 978 1 85775 755 2

Typeset by Anne Joshua & Associates, Oxford
Printed and bound by TJ International Ltd, Padstow, Cornwall

Contents

Foreword

It is with great pleasure that I write this foreword for *Religions, Culture and Healthcare: a practical handbook for use in healthcare environments*. In the Equality and Human Rights Group at the Department of Health, we actively promote innovative approaches to embedding the principles of equality, fair treatment, dignity and respect and valuing diversity into the Department and the NHS. These values and principles lie at the heart of the Department's drive to recognise the needs of patients and staff from diverse religious groups, and to respond sensitively and appropriately to those needs.

This is a much-welcomed guide on an issue which is at the heart of so many of us – our faith, our individual cultural identity, and our religious and spiritual needs. We are fortunate to live in a multi-cultural, multi-faith society, and the fact that the UK has more diverse faith communities than any other country in the European Union is something that we have every reason to be proud of. Valuing differences unites us, bringing us together and strengthening our society.

This guidance highlights the importance of celebrating this diversity as well as dealing with the challenges it poses us. It promotes a commitment to dignity and respect, to providing appropriate and sensitive care to all, and to patient-led care and individual choice at all stages of a patient's health and social care, from birth to the end of life.

It is a key part of the NHS Plan that any reform of the NHS and social care must ensure the delivery of fair, appropriate and equitable access of services to all. Indeed, the White Paper *Choosing Health*, published in November 2004, underlined our aim for everyone to achieve improved health, and to focus specifically on inequalities in health.

Spiritual care, then, is something that is essential within the NHS. As an organisation employing over 1.4 million staff, and with over five and a half million elective hospital admissions every year, it's vital that the NHS positions itself at the forefront of recognising the needs of the diverse patients and users that are part of, and use, its services.

We need to ensure that we are able to respond to the religious and spiritual needs of patients and staff, whatever their faith or belief. This is why I am delighted to write the foreword for this guidance which contributes towards making the NHS a place where people from all backgrounds feel valued, respected and treated fairly – a crucial goal for us all in delivering a patient-led NHS.

Surinder Sharma
National Director for Equality and Human Rights
Department of Health and the NHS
December 2005

Preface

All healthcare providers are required to have a sound working knowledge of the main religions to enable them to give sensitive and appropriate care to patients. This handbook is intended to be of practical assistance to healthcare staff in helping them to gain a fuller understanding of the nine world faiths and to be able to apply this knowledge in a variety of circumstances. I have also included information about some less well-known and some emerging faith communities as these also take their place within a society where diversity is the norm and no longer the exception. Collectively these faith communities represent a cultural and religious diversity that is vibrant and creative. Individually they present challenges to healthcare providers to develop and manage their services in ways that are more sensitive and responsive to their patients' particular needs.

A major precept in this book, both explicit and implicit, is the necessity for healthcare professionals to maintain an openness of mind – a positive regard – towards all patients, and to seek to avoid at all costs an easy placing of them within certain stereotypical frames. In this way the care that is provided can be of the highest order in relation to the patients' cultural, religious and spiritual needs and requirements. The information provided here could be regarded as a starting point on a journey of mutual discovery between the healthcare provider and the patient. On this journey into new territory there are highly significant clues to inform and improve not only the relationship between the healthcare professional and the patient, but also to improve the outcome of treatment.

The design of this handbook is intended to facilitate access to various types of information relating to the different stages and needs of life from within the spectrum of both major and minor religions. It is not intended that it should sit on a high shelf behind the locked doors of an office. Better that it is always to be found, increasingly dog-eared perhaps, at the nursing station, and in the pockets of doctors and other non-ward-based healthcare staff. Although it has been my intention to provide essential and relevant information, I have steered away from an encyclopaedic approach. I hope that as healthcare professionals gather this essential information they will also become confident in its judicious application, avoiding the stereotypical responses in order to discover the individual at the heart of their care. If additional information about certain aspects of patient care within a particular religion is needed, I hope that the Resources section at the end of the volume will provide further signposts for this journey.

Susan Hollins
December 2005

About the author

Susan Hollins BA (Hons), Cert Adv Psychodynamic Counselling has enjoyed a varied ministry since leaving university in the mid-1970s. She spent three years in South Africa within a Religious Community which was committed to racial justice. On her return to the UK, she trained for the Church's ministry at Lincoln Theological College, serving first of all in the Church in Wales, and then from 1988 to 1999 in the Diocese of Bristol (Church of England). She has served in a variety of parishes, latterly as Vicar of Longwell Green, Diocesan Ecumenical Officer and Honorary Canon of Bristol Cathedral. In 1999, Susan took up an appointment as healthcare chaplain within the NHS, working in the acute sector. Since autumn 2004, she has been working as one of four Lead Chaplains appointed by the NHS to take forward the modernisation agenda for spiritual healthcare.

Acknowledgements

Much of the information contained within this book is in the public domain, and is often passed on by word of mouth. My role therefore has been that of gatherer of scattered information. Other people have also been collecting this important information for use not only within healthcare, but also in business environments.

Particular thanks are due to the following: Dr Husna Ahmad, Mr Saif Ahmad and Revd John Evens of Faith Regen UK; Mark and Lynda Elding of the Pagan Federation; the Hospital Information Services of the Jehovah's Witnesses; Becky Lawson, Lead Nurse for Essence of Care Benchmarks, Barnet and Chase Farm NHS Trust; Mr Tony Lobl, Christian Science Committee on Publication, London.

Chapter 1

Cultural and religious diversity within healthcare

As societies become more diverse, so within healthcare increasing emphasis is rightly being given to the particular needs and requirements of the individual patient – not only in relation to their clinical needs, but also in relation to their cultural, religious and spiritual needs. Hospitals are places where people struggle to hang on to their individuality amid the clinical procedures set in place to make them physically or mentally well. Failing to pay proper attention to the individual – for example, taking the care to find out about their dietary requirements, whether they ascribe to any particular religion, how they would prefer to be addressed, etc. – only reinforces their vulnerability and a feeling that they are no longer in control of what happens to them.

We know that stereotypes reinforce negative thoughts about those who are different from ourselves, yet how often do we base our approach to patients upon such stereotypes? How often do we work from the foundation of our own assumptions and limited knowledge about other cultures and traditions when caring for patients? How often do our own prejudices lie hidden just below the surface of these narrow patterns of thinking? Such limited knowledge and understanding can only reduce the quality of care that we provide for those whose language and lifestyle is clearly different from our own. Yet if we were to be the patient in the bed, how might we feel if a healthcare professional was to treat us with the same narrowness of thinking and of approach and categorise us without bothering to discover the reality behind the stereotype?

We are cultural beings. From birth to death, culture informs and shapes us – for better as well as for worse. Every culture has its shadow side, which often emerges at points of personal or communal crisis, when we discover its limitations upon us. The positive elements of culture are often what we recall when we are far from what we recognise as our home and our roots, and when we crave the familiarity and comfort of what is normal and usual to us in terms of the food we eat, the language we use, the buildings that we live in, the things we enjoy doing, and so on. Between the crisis and the need for 'home comfort', culture is implicit in every part of our lives, so that sometimes we struggle to define what is culturally distinct about ourselves and the community that we call 'ours'. Sometimes definitions and critiques of our culture belong only to the comedian and the satirist, or to the travel writer – those who enjoy observing the oddities and richness of what is usual and ordinary and commenting upon them in their idiosyncratic ways that make us laugh or rage, or both. Within a society that is inherently diverse, we can no longer live as if the culture is monochrome. Even within societies that share a common heritage and language, there are cultural nuances and shifts, so that we are identified by our regional accents, the phrases that we use at particular times; the food that we eat in the different regions from which we come, and so on. These straightforward examples of cultural diversity illustrate a simple truth, namely that societies have been both threatened and strengthened by rich diversity throughout history. We also know, at great cost, that cultures and indeed whole peoples have been destroyed by an unbalanced desire on the part of others for a monochrome culture that can be controlled. Today in many countries there is a far greater diversity of people from very different cultures who seek to coexist creatively, and to build a future together. One of the essential characteristics of being part of such diverse societies is that each of us has a responsibility not only to understand our own culture, but also to know about and understand other cultures. We need to be both aware of and intelligent about our own culture, with its benefits and shortcomings, and at the same time to become far more literate about cultures different from our own. By engaging in a journey of discovery about other cultures, we will become more tolerant and understanding of others who are 'not like us'. Within healthcare environments, where patients are naturally vulnerable, our greater understanding and appreciation of different cultures will deepen our pastoral care as well as our clinical care.

In seeking to understand the different elements of culture, the image of an onion, with many different layers, has been used.[1] The different layers illustrate the ways in which culture influences our lives, from the implicit to the explicit. The outer layer illustrates how culture influences the externals of our lives, namely what is articulated in a variety of ways (e.g. what we say or do, how we dress, the food we eat, the design of the buildings in our towns, villages and cities). The second layer illustrates how culture informs and shapes the norms and values in our society and community. At this level the influences are, in the main, unspoken and implicit, tending towards universal themes relating, for example, to ethical standards and values – right and wrong, good and bad, and how people's behaviour reflects these values and ethics. The final, core layer contains those elements of culture whose threads can be traced through centuries of evolution and development and which focus upon the initial creation and foundation of a community, and a civilisation – the immediate environment, and the potential resources of climate and geography for the establishment and maintenance of a community/society. It is this deeply hidden element or layer of culture that provides the foundation for the other layers that emerge over time as the foundation, the first community, increases in strength and intelligence. This core element establishes and nourishes what Trompenaars refers to as the 'basic assumptions' of any culture,[2] which are deeply implicit and therefore not generally articulated.

Geert Hofstede, a Dutch cultural analyst,[1] has identified several levels of uniqueness in what he calls 'human mental programming'. These levels of uniqueness are *human nature* (the foundation layer), *culture* (the middle layer) and *personality* (the top layer). The programme or pattern also recognises and includes three other key elements that are pertinent to each level, namely the universal, that which is inherited, and that which is specific to an individual or group. The foundation level of human nature possesses universal characteristics such as needs and abilities, and the ability to feel and express – or withhold – emotion, alongside inherited characteristics that influence and modify these universal abilities. Likewise, culture is both learned and specific to a group or society. Because culture is learned, it is not only passed on from one generation to another but can also be passed to different groups. Within this programme or pattern an individual has the facility to absorb or embrace both the learned and the inherited ways of being and interacting in the world and with others, while at the same time possessing characteristics unique to that person. When we apply this understanding to cultural differences, there is every indication that a person can adapt successfully to different cultural patterns and traditions, as well as being able to move and to live easily within different cultures, belonging to more than one dominant cultural pattern.

Yet culture is only one element of many that inform and shape our identity. These elements can be viewed as fluid overlapping patterns (*see* Figure 1.1) rather than as static forms that do not interact with each other. From the moment of our birth we are shaped and formed by our experiences, which are set within a familial group, a neighbourhood, a society, a particular religion perhaps, a certain culture, a particular race, and so on.

When viewed in this way it becomes clear that any combination of these elements will provide the dominant strands in our sense of identity. Equally, the dominance of these elements will shift in relation to the different roles that we undertake on a daily basis. When a person is a hospital patient the pattern shifts once more, with identity being more focused upon physical and mental health and family relationships. Religion and spirituality may also increase in significance during this time.

Given this varied and shifting pattern, the application of stereotypes to those 'not like us' is highly inappropriate. When we attend with interest to just one of these elements, we enter the patient's own world and begin to see through their eyes. We become more able to perceive the appropriateness or inappropriateness of the care given to them.

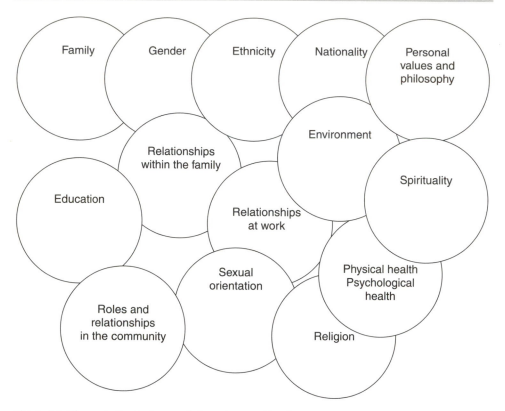

Figure 1.1 Elements that inform and shape human identity.

The questioning of patients about their physical habits and needs is necessary in hospital. Many intimate enquiries are made in order to enable treatment plans to be established. Yet of equal importance are the non-clinical questions that are often omitted because the member of staff either does not consider the matter sufficiently important or is too embarrassed to ask. For example, the question about a patient's religion is generally omitted on the grounds of embarrassment on the part of the healthcare worker, or because they do not consider such information to be significant to the overall care of the patient. In such circumstances it is essential for healthcare professionals to be able to set aside their personal beliefs and opinions in order to pay full attention to the patient, whose cultural needs and/or religious belief may be of profound significance and will be a major factor influencing their attitude to illness and their recovery. Another similar area of omission relates to the dietary needs of patients. If a patient is diabetic, the relevant box will be ticked. By contrast, this question arises infrequently if the patient's dietary requirements are influenced by their religious beliefs. Assumptions are often made about the person which lead to the wrong type of meals being served. For example, a female Jewish patient who exercised moderate discipline in relation to her diet was not eating the regular meals that were being provided, and as a consequence of this was very hungry. She had not wished to 'make a fuss' about the matter, and was trying her best to manage with the food provided. On the other hand, the staff had never asked her why most of her meals were being returned with little having been consumed. No one had offered her the kosher meal sheet. Was this because her name did not seem to be 'Jewish'?

Increasing numbers of people have multiple ethnic and cultural identities, and have a mixed heritage. In general, people manage to live with these differences and move smoothly between the different worlds that they represent. Particular care must be taken when making any note of a patient's ethnic identity. For example, it must not be assumed that because a patient is Asian he or she must therefore be Muslim. These kinds of assumptions only create further confusion. As different emphasis will be given by different people to the components of their cultural/ethnic identities in relation to different circumstances, this further reinforces the need for healthcare staff to be self-aware when caring for patients, in order to avoid putting people in unhelpful pigeonholes.

Much can be learned from people who belong to ethnic minority groups who have left behind the security of their own country with its particular habits and traditions and who have struggled to adapt to a new and very different culture. In the process of adaptation many such people become far more aware of their own culture as well as of the new culture. Sometimes this leads them to become more critically aware of the short-falls in their normative culture at the same time as being critical of the new culture which is often felt to be overwhelming. This experience is both costly and potentially creative.

A healthcare culture often threatens to dominate and overwhelm the individual patient and their family. This pattern is exacerbated when the culture and ethnic identity of the patient and their relatives is different from that of the country in which the healthcare takes place. Immense barriers, not least of language and interpretation, are erected, across which the easiest route to take is the 'normative' one, to the detriment of the patient's psychological well-being. Yet the dominant healthcare culture of a country may also threaten to overwhelm those for whom there are no immediate cultural differences of language. One reason for this is that being a patient in hospital can be both an alien experience and sometimes an alienating one. We are uprooted from all that is familiar in order to become dependent on both the healthcare professionals who treat us, and the treatment processes that are set in place for our recovery. Adjustment to this naturally takes time even when there are no significant cultural differences. It takes much longer, if it occurs at all, when the cultural differences are not recognised and supported. Another reason for the tendency of a healthcare culture to overwhelm those for whose well-being it is established is that the healthcare institution does not possess the capacity to listen to those whom it treats. As a consequence the institution becomes more inflexible in its attitude and approach, while those whom it treats lose trust in its commitment to their well-being.

Different cultural traditions also influence the way in which an individual will respond to illness and to treatment. Such responses are as conditioned as those relating to the way in which we dress and behave both at home and in public. Some will regard illness as having a spiritual dimension, sometimes received as a judgment or as 'cause and effect', and will seek spiritual guidance and support. Others will regard illness as being caused by a combination of several factors, such as lifestyle, environmental conditions or just 'bad luck'. It is appropriate to consider and take seriously the patient's value and/or belief system as an inherent element within their total care not only from the perspective of seeking to listen actively to them, but also in order to support them in tapping into their inner resources and other support networks in order to strengthen their pastoral and psychological well-being.

Equally, not everyone has the same attitude towards healthcare professionals. Whereas in western society healthcare staff, in particular doctors, are held in high regard and often treated with awe, in other cultures healthcare staff are regarded as equals, and sometimes as friends in whom one can confide. With such differences in approach and emphasis it is all the more important for healthcare staff to work towards a mutual understanding of roles and responsibilities with the patients in their care, and not to assume that the usual patterns (the status quo) are the most appropriate ones.

It is always useful, and often a sobering exercise, to place ourselves imaginatively in the 'shoes' of the patients for whom we care. By doing so we begin to perceive that what is usual for us in terms of, for example, modes of speech may actually have created immense difficulties of understanding and trust for the patient. We can go further than this and develop a mental checklist of good practice in our care of patients whose culture is very different from our own. Included in this checklist are obvious elements alongside others that might be more difficult to apply.

- Develop a good awareness and understanding of your own cultural patterns and assumptions, especially where these might inhibit your positive response to patients who have a different culture.
- Be aware that culture is fluid and organic rather than rigid and unchanging.
- Seek to listen to the patient with an open mind and with attentiveness.
- Seek to discover more about the patient's values, beliefs and culture and the ways in which these are important to them.
- Seek to avoid stereotypical thinking and responses.
- Be aware of the other elements that form and sustain a person's identity.
- Use information about a person's culture, religion, etc. judiciously

rather than applying it rigorously and without due regard for their individual preferences.

Any substantive attention to cultural and religious needs does not come without financial cost. New costs such as the provision of a good interpreting service, or making sure that sufficient female doctors are employed within a hospital, to take two obvious examples, need to be factored into any business planning for a healthcare service. However, the financial costs to the health provider will always be greater when culturally sensitive services are not provided (e.g. the cost of formal complaints), to which must also be added the psychological cost to the patients and their families. Other elements of cost will often remain hidden as they relate more to lack of well-being than to balance-sheets. These include the wasting of both staff and patient time and, above all, strong feelings of frustration, helplessness, disillusion, alienation and lack of trust on the part of the patient and their relatives. Collectively these costs signal poor outcomes for those whose physical health is already compromised.

The establishment of trust is crucially implicit in all relationships between healthcare staff and the patient. In caring for patients from different cultures the establishment of trust is absolutely essential, in order that those who have already been made vulnerable through illness are not set at greater disadvantage by being treated without consideration for their cultural needs. Those who are unfamiliar with a healthcare culture are, in general, far less inclined to make themselves heard – not because they might not have a sound cause, but because the institutional culture that prevails alienates rather than supports them.

The challenge to develop culturally sensitive services within healthcare invites the institution to engage both in attentive listening to these different voices and in collaborative creative thinking in order to see how the shape of services might be altered to accommodate different needs. The financial costs incurred in any modifications to services will be outweighed by the increase in mutual understanding and trust, which will have its own beneficial effect on the patient population.

Changes to services as outlined here are already taking place, particularly in community services. However, it is often the larger institutions that are more resistant to the need to make these significant modifications in substantive ways, despite the positive evidence in favour of such changes in community services.

The routes to such changes lead through the educational pathways for all healthcare staff, as well as in careful attention to detail in healthcare practice. This handbook will play its part well if, as a result of judiciously applying the information contained within it, staff gain an increased understanding of the different beliefs and practices contained within the faith groups, and in so doing pay greater attention to the religious and cultural needs and requirements of those in their care. The ground swell of increased understanding and awareness that will be generated by this will in turn influence the pattern of service provision such that major discrepancies can be redressed.

References

1 Hofstede G (1991) *Cultures and Organisations: software of the mind.* McGraw-Hill Book Company, London.
2 Trompenaars F (1993) *Riding the Waves of Culture: understanding cultural diversity in business.* Nicholas Brealey, London.

Chapter 2

Spiritual care

What does it mean to be spiritual? What is the place of religion within spiritual care? Where does 'spiritual' belong? What is 'spiritual care'? These are increasingly pertinent questions for the healthcare community as it seeks to engage more fully with this important but often neglected element of patient care. There are further equally pertinent questions. Is any spirituality and spiritual discipline only found within and belonging to religion? Does religion have the sole and prior 'ownership' of anything spiritual? Is it possible to have a spiritual life while not professing any religious allegiance or specific faith? What difference is there between spirituality and religion?

This chapter will begin to map some of the routes that have been taken so far, and which might be taken, in response to some of these questions. Yet the questions themselves (and their answers) belong very much within the public domain as well as within the domain of the main religions and of all who seek to engage with a spiritual life and to derive meaning and purpose for their lives through it.

But what does it mean to be spiritual? A dictionary definition of the word 'spiritual' presents us first with a non-specific concept: 'of or relating to, or affecting the human spirit as opposed to material or physical things.'[1] Secondly it offers us a more focused definition: 'of or relating to religion or religious belief.'[1] A dictionary definition of religion provides several linked responses: 'the belief in and worship of a superhuman controlling power, especially a personal God or gods; a particular system of faith and worship; a pursuit or interest.'[1] A religion is a system of faith and worship, both of which express spirituality. Each religion has its own characteristics and, at best, provides room and encouragement for the exploration and expression of a variety of spiritualities within the overall framework of the beliefs, traditions and practices of the faith. It must be emphasised that religion and a religious belief should never exclude spirituality and a spiritual discipline/framework. Conversely, it should never be assumed that because a person does not subscribe to a particular religion they do not have any spirituality or interest in seeking spiritual meaning for their life.

Although such definitions provide us with a starting point, some might regard them as unhelpful and limiting. However, we can ask the following question: 'What affects our spirit?'. We might begin to answer this question in terms of emotions as well as in terms of external factors that have a direct effect upon our lives, both practically and in relation to how we feel. We might also ask, in relation to this question, 'Who affects our spirit?'. Our response to this question will begin to engage us in a consideration of the significant relationships that we have had and still have, and how these relationships nourish our spirit and our sense of purpose, of belonging, and of meaning of our lives.

When considering what it means to be spiritual it is helpful to consider not only any particular religious belief that a person may have, but also other aspects of their life which they regard as important, such as their relationships, their work, and so on. Some people take a distinctly philosophical approach to life that excludes any reference to a power other than themselves. Examples of such an approach include atheism, existentialism and humanism. However, whether approached from the context of a religious faith, or from the context of a specific or general philosophical and existential understanding, the search for meaning and purpose in life is common to all and provides a foundation from which to start to frame a broader set of definitions for what we understand the term 'spiritual' to mean, and how spiritual care within healthcare environments might be formulated.

It is misleading to think that because the number of people who profess any form of religious faith and practice is, on the whole, dwindling in western society, an interest in and curiosity about a spiritual element to human existence is also declining. In contrast to the dwindling numbers of adherents to the mainstream religions, there has been no decline in interest in and curiosity about spiritual matters, even if these seem to focus on a wide variety of approaches, ranging from New Age belief systems to what have been termed 'human potential movements.'[2] Those whose curiosity does not take them into New Age or human potential movements often retain or initiate a new connection with a traditional religion, while not wishing to subscribe to a particular set of beliefs with its own disciplines and practices. Such people engage in what is known as 'supermarket religion' – taking from several religions those elements that have some meaning for them and which they can use as resources for conducting their lives.

Another misleading understanding is that western society has become essentially materialistic and secular. Apart from the increase in the number of people who are actively seeking to discover more about different spiritual disciplines and traditions, there has been no significant decline in the number of individuals who adhere to common religion. The 2001 Census figures indicate that the UK is 72% Christian. However, this figure will largely consist of those whose allegiance to the Christian faith is nominal. Although a spiritual or religious belief and practice is regarded as intensely private, despite the emphasis on supermarket religion, a belief is never entirely self-generated but emerges in relation not only to the person's disposition in terms of thought and feeling, but also to the prevailing and immediate context. Thus it is more accurate to talk in terms of a common religion rather than a private one. Common religion encompasses the less mainstream elements of belief and practice. Some aspects of common religion will have strong links with the orthodox beliefs of a particular religion, while others will be associated with other religious beliefs, or with practices dissociated from the belief system. Even within such a pattern there will be considerable variations in the beliefs, so that it becomes easier to think of these as being set within a very broad spectrum. This type of relationship with orthodox, mainstream religion is not restricted to the Christian tradition but can be found within other religions, although to a lesser degree.

Common religion encompasses such habits as requesting a baptism, wedding or a funeral from the local church. Within a healthcare setting this request is reformulated as requesting a chaplain to attend at a death or to officiate at an emergency baptism or a wedding. Another category that has been proposed is that of customary religion.[3] This term relates to a set of beliefs that still retains a connection, however loose, with the official teaching of the Roman Catholic Church. This will manifest itself in a healthcare setting as a request for the Roman Catholic Chaplain to provide 'Last Rites' (a sacramental ministry of anointing with holy oil and administering of Holy Communion), even though the patient has 'lapsed' over many years and may even have turned their back on the beliefs and practices of the faith. This represents one end of the broad spectrum of common or customary religion in which there are often strong links and associations with the Christian faith, its beliefs and its practices. At the other end of this spectrum may be found 'beliefs' and practices that are more commonly associated with superstition than with faith. These include healing, fate, luck, the paranormal, tarot cards and meditation, although this list is not exhaustive. Such practices and the belief patterns associated with them are not easily quantified or set within any clearly defined framework of belief, but they are frequently a very forceful element of a person's response to crisis. For example, a chronically ill patient may be in bed surrounded by artefacts and symbolic objects belonging to several faiths, and none, even though their faith has been given as Hindu.

Many people admit that they 'believe' but that they no longer 'belong' to a particular faith community. This reflects the 'supermarket' approach to religion, and is reminiscent of the thought which generated the line in an old hymn that 'one is nearer to God in a garden than any place on earth.' Membership of a faith community is now reduced to smaller numbers of the faithful who have to provide much of the financial support to maintain the viability and visibility of the community at a local level. However, this particular approach – to believe without actually belonging to one's faith community – is regarded as a status that is attained when a person does not make an active choice to pursue the Ariadne thread of curiosity, believing and belonging any further. The consequence is that such individuals are left without a framework for further enquiry and development, and tend to drift into other even more formless expressions and experiences of the spiritual and religious. This pattern is in line with the postmodern emphasis upon fragmentation and self-fulfilment – that from the fragments an individual should be able to construct for him- or herself a coherent belief system.

However, by contrast with the free-flowing individual approach to belief and belonging, there is another pattern of modern religious behaviour that moves in the opposite direction towards a reassertion of traditional beliefs, often with a robust fundamentalist element within them. Alternatively, one particular aspect of what has become fragmented is chosen and expanded to provide an overarching worldview. Conservatism within Christianity and Islam is very strong at the present time, and accounts for much that is in protest against what appear to be permissive and highly individuated cultural patterns. Yet such fundamentalism is also found within secular cultures and competes with its religious counterparts. Thus even at the other end of the spectrum of common religion there is a bewildering variety of beliefs and practices that are in active use within western society. Healthcare professionals must at least be aware of these nuances; so that when those who believe and practise in these varied ways become patients of a healthcare institution there is a readiness to avoid the easy stereotype and to begin to engage with the person.

Within the UK, despite the consistency in the level of common religion, alongside the increase in the number of people who are actively curious about a wide range of alternative and New Age beliefs, there is a general sense that anything connected with religion should be considered with reserve and some scepticism. Unlike the newly emergent spiritualities, the main religions carry an immense amount of negative 'baggage' that often skews the perceptions and responses of those who work in public-sector organisations. Those who are active members of a faith community, as well as those who represent such communities at local, regional and national levels, are often faced with negative responses based on the view that 'religion is harmful to health'. Religion is often blamed for a conservative approach to new socio-economic developments, and is perceived to be something of a fundamentalist killjoy. It is possible to say that all religions are hindered and significantly disadvantaged by those whose more overtly fundamentalist approach to life is often that which gains the attention of the general public. The moderate and wise voice within all of the main religions is barely heard, and when it is heard it is often derided. Such public opinion filters through to the healthcare environment, too. Healthcare chaplains, whose role is the spiritual, pastoral and religious care of patients, staff and relatives, often have that role curtailed as a direct consequence of this unfortunate perception that religion is related to only a small part of life and that, in general, religion is not particularly helpful or healthful.

This misconception might begin to be amended by careful consideration of what is sacred and what is secular. As the main religions seem to be removed from the realities of daily life rather than having direct relevance to the whole of life, so the New Age movements have gained some ascendancy, seeking to reclaim the whole of life as a sacred space in itself. The apparently consumerist society which seems to be prevalent in western countries exercises a certain ambivalence towards the sacred. Part of the reason for this is that the sacred is, on the whole, connected with the major religions and the diverse sacred spaces which are theirs – cathedrals, places of pilgrimage, holy temples, rivers, and so on.

Although many people do 'shop around' to find the various elements from different religions (old and new) for their spiritual shopping basket, the main Christian denominations have not excluded themselves from this approach to a spiritual life and discipline – many use marketing strategies to attract new believers.

Both alternative medicine and alternative spiritual paths have eschewed such approaches in favour of a strong emphasis upon what could loosely be called 'right relationship'. A right relationship in these circumstances involves the individual not only in seeking a healthful balance between their body, mind and spirit, and in their life as a whole, but also in their relationship with the natural world, and seeking to live harmoniously and healthfully within it. This is an organic approach to life that regards everything as sacred and as being in relationship, so that when one part of the 'body' is unhealthy, the whole body (the world) suffers.

New Age movements place great emphasis upon these varied but related elements of right relationship, seeking and working towards wholeness. Wholeness then becomes a spiritual concept that once more emphasises the sacredness of all life. New Age spirituality is, in general, distanced from traditional Christian belief and teaching, although the common thread to each is that the Christian traditions also place great emphasis upon wholeness and right relationship, but within the context of right relationship with God primarily, with all other relationships secondary to this. New Age philosophies are often seen as rivals of orthodox belief systems, especially since there is no pressure with regard to individual assent to a particular set of beliefs, which is often seen as a major advantage.

Ironically, as the relationship between the main religions and society in general has loosened, particularly in the UK, the sacred is not disappearing, but is emerging. Through the New Age philosophies the concept of the sacred has begun to move out into the common domain, and is no longer understood to be exclusive to the main religions. This shift could assist the emerging discussions within healthcare institutions with regard to a fuller understanding of spiritual care and how this care may be provided for all patients. As more people turn to unconventional, unorthodox spiritual pathways (and complementary medicine), so the 'marketplace' is open to fresh influences which have the potential to reframe the old arguments, tensions and proprietorial attitudes concerning what is spiritual and what is religious into a more expansive exploration. The latter should ideally be a joint venture between representatives of the main religions and those for whom a less well-trodden route is preferable.

From the perspective of a healthcare chaplain within the Christian tradition, I am looking for ways in which all those who are engaged in developing a spiritual framework for their life who also have a concern for the well-being of society can begin to reflect upon what it is to be spiritual, what it means to be religious, and how appropriate spiritual care can be developed within healthcare institutions. All who are concerned with the development of a spiritual life will have a major interest in this emerging element within patient care, with a view to providing care that is well constructed and balanced.

Theoretically there should not be any dichotomy between the practice of a religion and a spiritual life, although the quality of both will vary and will be dependent upon external factors such as the cultural environment, the freedom to observe one's religion, the size of the faith community, the personality of the individual concerned and the various influences upon them, as well as upon their personal preferences for particular aspects of their faith. As the earlier parts of this chapter have illustrated, a spiritual discipline/life may take many forms and have different emphases. Some of these emphases will overlap with concepts that are found in other areas, while some will belong only to a particular religion or spiritual movement.

It is important to stress that the main religions, as well as some of the newly emergent spiritual movements, have tremendous resources for the creation, nourishing and sustaining of a spiritual life – taproots reaching into deep wells whose foundations were set thousands of years ago. Yet it is also possible to say that spirituality, and a spiritual life, are not necessarily the preserve of the main religions, or indeed of any spiritual development movement. However, it is reasonable to assert that the search for a meaning and purpose for human existence is common to us all and is not the preserve of the religions and the religious. The form that this search and, hopefully, the discovery take is necessarily and significantly varied. It is also reasonable to assert that there are likely to be areas of commonality where the religious and the philosophical, alongside other approaches to life, have shared sets of meaning. Shared sets of meaning would include such things as the importance of relationship (with others, and with the past, the present and the future), the importance and significance of place, the importance of belonging and of contributing and giving to others, and the significance of loss.

It is possible to regard spirituality as being akin to a broad spectrum encompassing religious belief and practice, New Age movements and

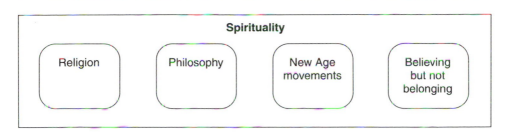

Figure 2.1 A spectrum for consideration of spirituality.

personal belief systems independent of any particular religious belief and practice (believing without belonging).

Disintegration – falling to pieces – is a reaction to a life crisis, whether this takes place at the point of impact, or is delayed for an unspecified length of time. Many people 'hold themselves together' at the time of crisis and later, when the crisis is over, they allow themselves to 'fall apart' to some extent. In crisis our response is often that of 'fight or flight', when the adrenalin rush sometimes makes it difficult to respond more rationally. One of the purposes of spiritual care, whether at a time of crisis or over a much longer period of time, is to facilitate the individual's response and to support them in articulating their deeper thoughts and feelings. This can be summed up in terms of a search for integration – to seek for and find purpose and meaning in circumstances that often feel devoid of all meaning. Whether or not this integrative work takes place within the framework of a particular religion will depend upon the individual but, as Figure 2.1 shows, the backdrop for all of the different approaches to life (and the diagram is not necessarily comprehensive) is that of a spiritual search and expression which allows for a richly varied set of responses from one or several of the different sub-sets.

A word of caution is needed at this point. Throughout any developmental process that involves cultivating and sustaining a more thoroughly comprehensive understanding of spirituality and spiritual care within a healthcare environment, it is important not to create overarching systems which attempt in a universal manner to embrace all that can be understood about spirituality and spiritual care. Allowance must be made for variation and diversity of expression and the provision of a service both within and across the different religious and ethnic groups.

Historically the spiritual, religious and pastoral care of patients, staff and relatives in hospitals has been the domain of the hospital chaplaincy, which has been staffed by Christian ministers representative of the mainstream denominations. In practice these have tended to be Anglican priests, with more specific provision made for Roman Catholic patients. Healthcare chaplaincy works from a broad pastoral foundation whereby spiritual and religious care is provided for any who request it for themselves or who have been referred to the chaplaincy service.

A person does not have to subscribe to a particular religion in order to receive pastoral and spiritual support from healthcare chaplains. This approach reflects the broad spectrum of spirituality shown in Figure 2.1 and the common areas outlined in relation to a search for meaning. Chaplains are able to provide spiritual care in appropriate and diverse ways for those who express distress and need.

With the increasing cultural and religious diversity within the UK and other western countries, healthcare chaplaincy has committed itself to working more closely with representatives of other major faiths in the spiritual, religious and pastoral care of patients, relatives and staff. Although the practice of Christian pastoral and sacramental care is broad-based, there are limitations to this with regard to patients from other faiths for whom the ministrations of a Christian minister would be inappropriate. As each religion understands and exercises pastoral and religious care in different ways, care must be taken not to adopt a 'one-size-fits-all' approach to such a delicate area of healthcare.

Each of the main religions has a different concept of what it means to be spiritual – to have a spiritual life or spirituality. This is in contrast to emerging constructs for spirituality, which tend to oversimplify. Within the USA the work of Larry and Lauri Fahlberg and of Pamela Reed exemplifies such approaches, which are not necessarily relevant to people who belong to the major faiths who have very different under-standings of what spiritual care means, and for whom even the concept of 'pastoral care' is unusual. This emerging but overarching definition of spiritual care is closest to but not wholly aligned with Christian models. There are three main elements to this understanding of the nature of spiritual care. The first is an emphasis on holistic care, which considers the individual's feelings and any beliefs or philosophical framework for living. The second element is an emphasis on the search for and discovery of meaning that can be articulated through beliefs and values. The third element is an emphasis on a 'capacity for self-transcendence that is expressed by expanding personal boundaries intrapersonally, interperson-ally and transpersonally – inward, outward and upward. Transcendence can be found within or beyond self, depending upon one's religious or philosophical beliefs.'[4]

It has been asserted by Ian Markham[5] that this definition of spirituality is a secular version of the Christian understanding of spirituality. Such a definition is reductionist in its approach, watering down the essential elements of orthodox concepts of spirituality from within Christianity. Although such reduced concepts of spirituality might be understood, if not accepted, by the Christian traditions, they are certainly unacceptable to those who subscribe to other major faiths, on the basis that these have a very different understanding of spirituality.

In the previous chapter I emphasised the necessity for healthcare providers to take diversity seriously rather than to seek to develop uniform systems that only pay tacit attention to the creative differences between cultures and religions. This is no less important when we consider the detail of the theological understanding that each major faith has in relation to the care of those who are ill and in distress, how each of these religions understands the predominantly Christian notion of pastoral care, and how relevant and significant each of the religions considers this to be.

However, when we consider briefly the notion of transcendence it is clear that this is a foreign concept to most of the major faiths. The spirituality of Islam emphasises the extinction of the self in Allah. This is not to be considered negatively but revered, for the purpose of the self is for it to merge with God. By contrast, Judaism emphasises the discovery of that which is spiritual within everyday life. This to some extent explains the food laws and other disciplines that practising Jewish people exercise, for they are reminders of the presence of God and of the 'transcendent significance'[4] of the normal and everyday. Hinduism does not really have a concept of transcendence, as it emphasises that the divine is within each individual. The task of each person is to make an inward journey and in so doing to encounter the divine – the cosmic self (Brahman). The Buddhist emphasis, by way of further contrast, is on the transience of all things and on ethical (right) living: 'Spirituality, then, is the cultivation of certain dispositions that integrate this awareness of the transient nature of all things into one's life.'[5]

There is an understandable reserve within the faith communities about the apparent ease with which any definition of spirituality can be developed for use within healthcare contexts. Each religion naturally exercises a different understanding of spirituality and its expression, so how can such diversity be encapsulated within one or two sentences? Another justifiable concern is that since spirituality is at the heart of the faiths, it is important first for this to be acknowledged and understood by healthcare providers, and for there to be strong encouragement to include a fuller understanding of the different religions within all training programmes for healthcare staff. Secondly, it would be important to engage members of different religious groups in a creative and ongoing debate about what is meant by spirituality and spiritual care within secular contexts, and for this debate also to be included within training programmes. One element of any dialogue such as this would be to explore whether spirituality can be identified and developed apart from any religion, and if so, what the characteristics might be. My earlier reflections in this chapter indicate that it is possible to discern an initial framework for understanding spirituality apart from a religious framework by considering existential themes, such as a search for meaning and belonging, or the importance and meaning of different kinds of relationship. However, such a definition might not encompass all that might be considered for such an important subject. At present there are religious definitions of spirituality and there are also some secular/philosophical definitions, but each operates within separate areas. The Christian traditions have developed and provided leadership within healthcare chaplaincy (spiritual health-care) alongside their Jewish colleagues for many years, and representatives from the other major faiths are now joining them. Alongside an increasing understanding of spiritual care from within the religions, the nursing communities have also provided a seedbed for some secular and philosophical concepts of spirituality and spiritual care. These have also found their way into the arena of healthcare chaplaincy and have generated some interesting developments in spiritual care. However, much more dialogue between these two communities is essential in order to gain deeper understanding from the resources that are available and for this understanding to be disseminated widely and become an implicit part of the training programme of any healthcare professional.

Although it is tempting to approach this subject with the intention of reducing it to the lowest common denominator, this temptation must be avoided, not least because the subject itself – what it means to be spiritual, what spirituality means, the significance of religion – is too complex to be so readily simplified. Any worthwhile and continuing dialogue about spirituality, which in itself is metaphysical rather than scientific, will undoubtedly be concerned with what it means to be a person, and this in turn will involve further reflection on the purpose and action of a person both in relationship to others, and in society.

In any serious consideration of both cultural diversity and spiritual care within healthcare provision, it becomes evident that we have embarked upon what might be termed a reclamation of the individual – a creative recognition of the person who is at the heart of any treatment. This recognition naturally leads to further reflection upon what it means to be a person. It also leads to the posing of searching questions concerned with deeper understandings of religion and spirituality and how these inform and influence the person for whom we have a professional responsibility – whether as doctor, chaplain, nurse, porter, therapist, etc. Above all I hope that these searching challenges will lead all of us within healthcare to consider together some of the potential solutions, for the benefit of all.

In this chapter I have merely begun to outline some of the elements that will be found within any consideration of an understanding of a spiritual life, what it means to be religious, and what it means to maintain and nourish spirituality, as well as considering how the divisions between what is regarded as secular and sacred are shifting. Within the overall context of cultural diversity the time has come to begin to address these other significant elements of diversity that reflect and give clues about what it means to be a person. These 'clues' can no longer be reduced or disregarded by healthcare institutions as being peripheral to the well-being of patients. In addition, the increasing emphasis on patient and public involvement in the way that health services are configured and provided offers another forum in which this important dialogue may take place, where the diverse voices of patients and public can be heard, and received.

Within healthcare chaplaincy/spiritual healthcare these dialogues are already taking place, yet they are often peripheral to the very institution that they concern. Although some may regard religion as being damaging to health (and there is strong evidence to support this view, just as there is strong evidence to support its beneficial influence on health), nevertheless the vast knowledge and experience that the main religions possess both individually and collectively in relation to concepts of 'right living' (a balanced life) as well as in relation to the care of the sick and the dying must not be either derided or ignored as being irrelevant to the age in which we live.

There are many potentially enriching and influential dialogues and exchanges that must begin to be established at every level within healthcare with the aim of developing healthcare services which are more culturally and spiritually intelligent. Such dialogues and decisions will be implicitly complex and must not only involve the different professional communities within healthcare, but also the general public for whose health and well-being the services are designed and established.

References

1 Pearsall J (ed.) (2001) *The Concise Oxford Dictionary* (10e revised). This edition published by BCA by arrangement with Oxford University Press, Oxford.
2 Davie G (1998) Faith and belief: a sociological perspective. Reprinted from Cobb M and Robshaw V (eds) *The Spiritual Challenge of Healthcare*, p. 92, with permission from Elsevier.
3 Hornsby-Smith M (1991) *Roman Catholic Beliefs in England.* Cambridge University Press, Cambridge.
4 Reed P (1998) The enchantment of healthcare: a paradigm of spirituality. Reprinted from Cobb M and Robshaw V (eds) *The Spiritual Challenge of Healthcare*, p. 42, with permission from Elsevier.
5 Markham I (1998) Spirituality and world faiths. Reprinted from Cobb M and Robshaw V (eds) *The Spiritual Challenge of Healthcare*, p. 77, with permission from Elsevier.

Chapter 3

Elements of care

For ease of reference, each section in Chapter 4 has a similar layout relating to the following areas:

- background and beliefs
- names
- religious obligations
- diet
- dress
- language
- birth
- personal hygiene
- gender, privacy and dignity
- attitude to illness
- blood transfusions
- contraception
- fertility treatment
- visiting
- dying and death
- post-mortem
- organ and tissue donation.

Religions and other faith groups within the United Kingdom

- Baha'i
- Buddhist
- Christian
- Other groups
  - Christian Science
  - Jehovah's Witness
  - Mormon (Church of Jesus Christ of Latter-Day Saints)
  - Rastafarian
- Hindu
- Islam
- Jain
- Jewish
- Pagan
- Sikh
- Zoroastrian

Baha'i

Background and beliefs

- The Baha'i faith was founded in Persia in 1844 by Husayn Ali, known to Baha'is as Baha'u'llah (Glory of God). It was declared as a new religion, different to Shia Islam practised in Iran.
- Four of the twelve key beliefs are as follows:
  - belief in one God
  - the unity of mankind
  - independent investigation of truth
  - the common foundation of all religions.
- Unity is a central theme of the Baha'i faith. Baha'is believe that there has only ever been one religion and one God, although people have called him by different names. Baha'is believe that Baha'u'llah was the great messenger who would bring peace to the world.
- Baha'is have a great respect for life. Each person has a soul that comes into being at conception. During a person's lifetime, the soul acquires spiritual attributes required for the next stage of existence, which occurs at death.
- The Baha'i faith is an independent world religion with its own laws and ordinances.
- Baha'is have a great respect for doctors and are encouraged to consult the best possible medical advice when ill.

Names

The manner of addressing the person will be influenced by their ethnic origin.

Religious obligations

There are three obligatory daily prayers, of which one must be said. Baha'is turn in the direction of Bahji in Israel – the burial place of Baha'u'llah.

Diet

- There are no dietary restrictions. Some Baha'is may be vegetarian, but this is not a religious requirement. Habit-forming drugs are forbidden.
- Fasting takes place each year during the holy season from 2 to 20 March. This is a time of spiritual regeneration. From sunrise to sunset each day Baha'is fast. During sickness, pregnancy and menstruation the

fast is lifted. Mothers who are breastfeeding, and people under 15 years or over 70 years of age are exempted from fasting.

Dress

In general there are no religious obligations with regard to everyday wear.

Language

Baha'i is an ethnically diverse religion. Baha'i families in the UK may speak several languages other than English, depending on their cultural background.

Birth

The birth of a child is a time of joy. There are no rituals associated with birth.

Personal hygiene

Baha'is require no special conditions with regard to washing, bathing, etc. Some may wish to wash before their daily prayer.

Gender, privacy and dignity

Baha'is do not object to being examined by doctors of the opposite sex.

Attitude to illness

Baha'is have great respect for scientifically-based medical opinion, and they are encouraged to seek out and comply with the best advice. Alongside medication the Baha'is also strongly believe in the power of prayer in the healing process.

Blood transfusions

Baha'is have no objection to blood transfusions.

Contraception

Family planning is left to the personal conscience of the Baha'i, but the following considerations should be borne in mind.

- Sterilisation in either sex is strongly discouraged. In cases where a medical condition is relevant to the decision, the individual should seek qualified advice.
- Methods of contraception that prevent implantation of the fertilised ovum are unacceptable, as Baha'is believe that the soul comes into being at conception.

Fertility treatment

Baha'is will make decisions relating to fertility treatment on an individual basis, with the underlying commitment to the sustaining of life.

Visiting

Baha'is will welcome visits by members of their local Spiritual Assembly.

Dying and death

- The body of a person is believed to be a vehicle of the soul, so Baha'is treat the body of a deceased person with great respect.
- The relatives or friends of Baha'is will wish to say prayers for the dead.
- Baha'i law prescribes that burial should take place at a distance of not more than one hour's journey from the place of death.
- Funerals are normally arranged by the family of the deceased if available, or on occasion by the Spiritual Assembly.

Post-mortem

There are no objections to post-mortems.

Organ and tissue donation

- Baha'is may leave their bodies for scientific research.
- Baha'is may donate organs and/or tissue for transplantation.

Buddhist

Background and beliefs

- This is the way of life for the people who follow the teachings of Buddha. The faith focuses on Mahatma Gautam Shakyamuni Buddha, who lived in India over 2500 years ago. He is worshipped not as a god, but as the founder of a way of life. Buddha is believed to have found the middle way between luxuries and asceticism. This is called the Eightfold Path to enlightenment, which is symbolised by an eight-spoked wheel.
- Buddhism is a highly individual spiritual path, as the religion has no single creed, authority or sacred book.
- Buddhism exists in a variety of forms, adapting itself to the cultures and peoples that engage in it.
- There are about 50 000 Buddhists within the UK, as well as numerous groups and sects around the world.
- Buddhism does not have a belief system. Its emphasis is upon teachings used as guides in daily life. The Five Precepts are the basic rules for daily living for lay Buddhists, and are concerned with refraining from:
  - harming living beings
  - taking what is not given
  - sexual misconduct and misuse of the senses
  - harmful speech
  - drink or drugs which could cloud the mind.
- Buddhists find support in the Buddha, in his teachings and in the community of Buddhists. They strive to live skilfully – that is, following the Buddhist precepts and teachings, being mindful of the effect of their behaviour upon others, and leading a peaceful existence that values humility. Ethical thinking and right actions are also important.
- Central to the Buddhist belief is the injunction not to cause harm to others, and to help all beings.
- The Buddhist aim is to achieve Nirvana – that is, a state of liberation characterised by freedom from suffering, death and rebirth.
- Buddhists believe in rebirth (not reincarnation), and believe that their actions in this life will affect the quality of the next. Therefore they accept all responsibility for their actions.

Names

- It is usual for Buddhists to have two or more names, the first of which may be the family name, and the second or subsequent name(s) the given name(s).

- It is advisable to ask first for the family name, and to use this as the surname.

Religious obligations

- Buddhist religious practice is very variable, depending upon the individual. It may include chanting and meditation.
- A peaceful environment is generally helpful.

Diet

- Diet varies according to the climate of the country. Generally speaking, Buddhists are vegetarian, as the notion of non-harm is central to Buddhist teaching.
- Salt-free salads, rice, vegetables and fruit are generally acceptable foods.
- Ordained and strict Buddhists may be vegan and may choose not to eat after midday. A modest diet signifies awareness that people generally eat more than they need.
- Fasting is neither a feature nor a practice among most Buddhists, with the exception of monks and nuns. Most fasting takes place on New Moon and Full Moon days, but there are also other festival days (e.g. Buddha's birthday, his death day, his enlightenment, his first sermon, and others).

Dress

- Generally there are no religious requirements concerning forms of everyday dress for lay Buddhists.
- Ordained monks and nuns are distinguished by their brightly coloured robes.

Language

Buddhist families in the UK may speak several languages other than English, including Tibetan, Cantonese, Hakka, Japanese and Sinhalese.

Birth

- A peaceful birth environment will be appreciated.
- No special ceremonies are required. A blessing may be performed later.

Personal hygiene

- There are no special obligations, but the following may be required:

- a container of water for washing if the toilet is separate from the bathroom
- showers are preferable to baths.
- Buddhists from different parts of the world may follow various social customs.

Gender, privacy and dignity

- There are no special obligations.
- Buddhist monks or nuns will prefer to be treated by a member of staff of the same sex. They may also have specific needs related to their vows.

Attitude to illness

- Helping people is fundamental to Buddhist ideas, so Buddhists will respect the medical staff for their help.
- Illness and suffering will be understood in relation to the Four Noble Truths:
  - the truth of suffering
  - the truth of the cause of suffering
  - the truth of the cessation of suffering
  - the Eightfold Path.
- Buddhists may prefer to maintain a clear mind when terminally ill. This may involve the refusal of pain-relieving drugs if these would impair mental alertness.
- Buddhists may traditionally and culturally favour the use of home remedies.

Blood transfusions

- There are no religious objections to blood transfusions.
- Buddhists generally regard the donation of blood an excellent means of giving to someone else.

Contraception

- This is not a cause of concern to Buddhists, who would usually practise any of the conventional methods.
- Any method of contraception that is used should be one which safe-guards the normal development of the baby if conceived
- Most Buddhists would not consent to an abortion because it would compromise the sanctity of all living beings.

Fertility treatment

The Five Precepts (and other beliefs) will provide the framework for all decisions relating to fertility treatment. Therefore it is important to attend to the individual's approach in the light of these beliefs.

Visiting

- Buddhist patients may welcome visits by other members of the local Buddhist community.
- Patients may require the help of a chaplain in arranging a time at which meditation may take place.

Dying and death

- Most Buddhists will provide medical staff with the name of the person to contact in the event of their death if this differs from their next of kin/ named person.
- The death of a person is viewed as a very important time. The body should be treated with the greatest care and respect, and it should be disturbed only for special reasons and with appropriate care.
- Buddhists regard the preparation for death as crucially important. This overrides any rituals associated with death.
- There is no single Buddhist ritual before, at the time of or after death. Examples of some practices are listed below.
  - A Buddhist priest or monk of the same school of Buddhism could be informed immediately so that prayers may be recited as soon as possible after the death.
  - Relatives/friends may wish the body to remain where it is until a priest is able to attend.
  - Sufficient time will be required for the prayers to be said.
  - It may not always be necessary for the priest to be present to recite prayers that may be recited at a distance (e.g. in a temple).
  - In some traditions it is customary for the body to remain at the place of death for up to 7 days to allow rebirth to take place. However, it is unusual for this practice to be enforced by relatives within a healthcare setting, although healthcare staff need to be aware of this practice.
- Buddhists generally prefer cremation to burial, as it is a symbol of the impermanence of the body.

Post-mortem

There are no objections to post-mortems.

Organ and tissue donation

- In Buddhism there are no injunctions for or against organ donation. Central to Buddhism is a wish to relieve suffering, and there may be circumstances in which organ donation may be seen as an act of charity.
- Each decision will depend upon the feelings of those involved and the teachings of the different schools of Buddhism.

Christian

Background and beliefs

Christianity begins with the person of Jesus Christ, who lived over 2000 years ago, and whom Christians believe to be both divine and human. Christians understand God to be one being, but revealed in three 'persons' – Father, Son and Holy Spirit. God is believed to have revealed himself through and in the life, death and resurrection of Jesus Christ.

Christians believe that God's forgiveness and healing extend to all people through the self-offering/sacrifice of Jesus Christ on the cross. Christians believe that through the death of Christ death itself has been overcome and that eternal life, which spans both earthly and spiritual worlds, is a gift of God to all in Christ.

The Church is the community of the faithful (i.e. believers), whose worship and service of God in the world extend his kingdom of love, truth, justice and peace. Christians believe in living according to the loving nature of God as revealed by Jesus' life and death, helped in this task by the Holy Spirit, and by communicating with God through prayer.

Sunday is the usual day for Christian worship because it is believed to be the day of the week on which Jesus was raised from the dead.

Christianity and its practice are very diverse, with many cultural/ ethnic influences upon worship and everyday life. There are many denominations, each with its own particular ethos and religious/ethical obligations.

Christian denominations

Church of England/Anglican

- Patients who choose this designation vary widely in their religious practice and requirements.
- Patients listed as Church of England may also be termed Anglican. The Church of England, the Church in Wales, the Church of Ireland and the Episcopal Church in Scotland are all part of the same Anglican family of churches worldwide.

Roman Catholic

Patients listed as Roman Catholic are part of the worldwide Roman Catholic Church.

Free Church

This is an umbrella term for a group of different denominations which include the following:
- Church of Christ
- Church of the Nazarene
- Congregational
- Free Church of England
- Free Evangelical Churches
- House Churches
- Independent Churches and Missions
- Independent Methodist
- Lutheran
- Pentecostal Churches
- Plymouth Brethren
- Salvation Army
- The Religious Society of Friends (Quakers)
- Baptist Church
- Methodist Church
- Moravian Church
- New Church
- Presbyterian Church/Church of Scotland
- Seventh-Day Adventist Church
- United Reform Church.

Orthodox

There are two traditions within Christian Orthodoxy, namely Greek and Russian. Coptic Christianity has strong links with the Greek orthodox tradition. Today Orthodox Christians belonging to one of these traditions may be found in Ethiopia, Serbia, Greece, Cyprus, Russia, Turkey and the UK. Religion is a predominant characteristic of Greek national identity, particularly among the ex-patriot communities.

Christian Science, Jehovah's Witness, Mormon (Church of Jesus Christ of Latter-Day Saints) and Rastafarian

- Each of these faith communities is distinct from mainstream Christianity in its origins, beliefs, practice and ethos, and functions autonomously apart from the networks binding the main denominations. However, some bonds, patterns and associations with certain aspects of the Christian faith are retained by each of these communities.
- Taking into account this belief differential, it nevertheless seems appropriate to include them within the broad remit of the Christian heading while providing a special section for each of them in which to set out their respective backgrounds and requirements.

General information

Names

- The term 'Christian name' refers to the first name that a person is given at their baptism. Historically a person who became a Christian during adulthood would receive a new 'baptismal' name to signify their new life in Christ.
- Nowadays the Christian name usually refers to the forename of a person that is followed by a family name. It is advisable to ask for the surname first and then for the other name(s).

Religious obligations

- Advent, Christmas, Ash Wednesday, Lent, Easter, Ascension Day and Pentecost are the major holy seasons of the Church, when attendance at church or chapel is expected.
- Within the different denominations there is a wide variety of religious practice.
- Prayer is important for Christians, who are encouraged to develop their own pattern and discipline that includes private devotion and attending public worship at church. Staff should respect the patient's need for quietness and privacy for their own prayers.
- Christians may welcome the opportunity to receive the sacrament of Holy Communion while they are hospitalised as inpatients.
- They may also welcome the opportunity to receive anointing and the laying on of hands for healing.
- Details of the requirements for particular denominations are provided under specific headings later in this chapter.

Diet

- Generally Christians are not forbidden to eat any particular kinds of foods.
- Some Christian denominations and other smaller Christian groups ban the use of stimulating substances (e.g. alcohol, tea, coffee) altogether.
- Ash Wednesday, which marks the beginning of Lent in February or March, is a customary day of fasting.
- Some Christians may observe the six-week period of Lent by refraining from consuming certain foods and/or drink (e.g. biscuits, chocolate, alcohol).
- Some Christians may wish to fast before receiving Holy Communion.

Dress

- In general, Christians are not obliged to dress in any particular way in terms of everyday wear.
- Monks or nuns may have forms of dress which would include the wearing of darker colours, full-length robes and (for women) head coverings.

Language

Christianity is ethnically diverse, and members of Christian families in the UK may speak several languages other than English, depending on their cultural background

Birth

- For many Christians it is important for a baby to be baptised/christened.
- Members of the Baptist Church (and small Christian groups) do not practise infant baptism and may prefer a service of blessing.
- If a baby is near to death an emergency baptism may be performed by the Healthcare Chaplain, by a local Christian minister known to the family, or by a nurse.
- The baptism of a dead baby is not usual practice.
- A service of blessing may be offered either at the time of death or shortly thereafter.

Personal hygiene

There are no special obligations with regard to hygiene for religious reasons. Be led by the individual patient.

Gender, privacy and dignity

In general, there are no special obligations on religious grounds. However, there will be variations within each denomination, so it is best to be led by the individual patient.

Attitude to illness

- Christian teaching encourages the faithful to respond to their illness as positively as possible, entrusting themselves to the healing and care of God in Jesus Christ.
- Christians will generally welcome the opportunity to receive Holy Communion.

- In addition, some may wish to make their confession to a priest.
- Anointing with holy oil, and the laying on of hands for healing, may also be required, especially at times of crisis.
- Privacy will be needed for all of these special services at the bedside.
- Terminally ill patients may welcome the opportunity to prepare themselves for death by means of prayers with a hospital chaplain/ local minister known to them.

Blood transfusions

In keeping with the self-giving love demonstrated by Jesus, Christians have no religious objections to transfusions.

Contraception

- Most Christian denominations allow people to make autonomous decisions within the context of their faith, recognising that contraception is a matter of individual responsibility.
- The official statement of the Roman Catholic Church is that contraception is not permitted. However, many couples within this denomination now make autonomous decisions about this practice.

Fertility treatment

In general, fertility treatment is supported, as it would be consistent with theological principles. However, it is important to be aware of individual circumstances which often prove to be the exception to general principles.

Visiting

- Within a framework of pastoral and spiritual care, chaplaincy staff are responsive to the patient's specific pastoral needs, whether or not these are clearly religious.
- Chaplains visit wards regularly and also respond to specific requests/ referrals made by the patient, their relatives or members of staff.

Dying and death

- It is good practice to anticipate the religious requirements of a patient who is dying, rather than leaving those requirements until the last moment.
- Patients or their relatives may ask for a chaplain to visit.
- If a patient or their relatives have not asked for this, staff can suggest that a chaplain visits.

- The chaplain will attend the patient in order to listen and to offer appropriate pastoral and religious support (e.g. prayers, anointing with oil).
- When a patient has died, the chaplain may still attend to say prayers, to support the relatives and to collaborate with other staff in doing so.

Post-mortem

There are no objections to post-mortems.

Organ and tissue donation

- Enabling life to be lived as fully as possible is consistent with the teachings of Jesus Christ.
- Christians are encouraged to help others in need. Discussing organ donation with the patient's family and friends is a responsible and thoughtful act.

Specific information for each denomination

Church of England/Anglican

- All confirmed members of the Church of England are eligible to receive Holy Communion, whether or not they are currently connected with a local church. Patients may derive particular comfort from Holy Communion which is administered by a chaplain at the bedside.
- Patients may wish to set aside time for private prayer without being disturbed, especially if their hospitalisation coincides with a major Christian festival, such as Christmas or Easter.
- Patients may wish a chaplain to pray with them and/or to provide the Sacrament of Anointing of the Sick/the laying on of hands for healing.
- Bereaved patients who are unable to attend the funeral may welcome the provision of a parallel funeral service by the chaplain at the bedside or in a quiet room.
- Patients may wish a chaplain to pronounce a blessing at certain times (e.g. after a civil marriage service performed by a Registrar within the hospital, on a wedding anniversary, or after psychic disturbance).

Dying and death

- Patients may wish the chaplain to visit them while they are dying in order to pray with them, commending them to the care and love of God.
- Some patients may wish to receive the Sacrament of Holy Communion before they die, if this is physically possible.

- Some patients may wish to receive the Sacrament of Anointing of the Sick.

Roman Catholic

A person's spiritual and religious needs will be dependent upon their particular circumstances. However, within the Roman Catholic Church there are certain expectations and obligations that may need to be fulfilled.

- To attend Mass on Sundays and Holy Days. Patients and their relatives welcome the opportunity to attend Mass in the hospital chapel.
- To receive Holy Communion: If a patient is unable to attend Mass, Holy Communion (the Sacrament) can be brought to them by the Roman Catholic Chaplain, by one of the Roman Catholic on-call chaplains or by a lay Eucharistic Minister.
- To receive a blessing or a visit from a chaplain
- To celebrate the Sacrament of Reconciliation (Confession). Patients may wish to make their confession to a priest in confidence and to receive absolution (God's forgiveness).
- To celebrate the Sacrament of the Sick. In the case of serious illness, major surgery or other times of crisis, the priest may administer this sacrament. It includes a Bible reading, the laying on of hands for healing, and anointing the person with holy oil.
- Patients may request help in their prayer, or ask for a Bible/rosary beads/prayer cards, etc.

Dying and death

- Patients may require the Roman Catholic chaplain to recite the Prayers for the Dying, commending the person to God, and assuring them and their relatives of God's love.
- When the patient has died, the chaplain will recite the Prayers for the Dead.
- Sometimes Roman Catholics from an older tradition, or those who are not too involved in the church, will ask for a chaplain to perform 'The Last Rites' for a seriously ill relative. There is actually no ceremony with this name. What is actually being asked for is a 'rite of passage' that could include the Sacrament of the Sick (Holy Communion) along with Prayers for the Dying or Prayers for the Dead.
- Catholic teaching encourages the participation of the church at all stages of illness, rather than only involving the priest at the very end.
- Staff who care for Roman Catholic patients should inform and assure them that the chaplain is there to provide help and support.

Free Church

- There will be a diversity of responses, depending upon the individual's usual practice. However, their practice may not differ greatly from that of a member of the Church of England.
- Patients may wish to receive Holy Communion.
- Patients may welcome the provision of the Sacrament of Anointing of the Sick/the laying on of hands for healing.
- Patients may request the chaplain to provide pastoral and spiritual support at a time of crisis.

Dying and death

- Within these denominations there is a wide variation depending upon the person's usual practice.
- Patients may require sacramental care similar to that given to Roman Catholic and Church of England patients.

Orthodox

Orthodox Christians belonging either to the Greek or the Russian Orthodox Church may be found in Ethiopia, and other parts of Africa, the Middle East, Bosnia, Serbia, Greece, Russia, Turkey and the United Kingdom.

Names

- Many children are named after their grandparents, as a sign of respect, and many Greek Orthodox names have their roots in the Christian Bible.
- Older members of the community may be addressed as Mr or Mrs, followed by their first name (e.g. Mr Andreas, Mrs Eleni).

Diet

- There are no dietary restrictions except during periods of fasting, when a person will abstain from eating animal or dairy products.
- Fasting takes place during Lent and Advent, before taking Holy Communion, and at certain other festivals.

Language

Most Orthodox Christian patients will speak English. Other languages will include Greek, Russian, Serbian, Amharic (Ethiopia) and Turkish.

Birth

- Babies are baptised soon after birth and become members of the Orthodox Church.
- In emergencies it will be appropriate for a baby to be baptised as quickly as possible by a member of the Orthodox Church.

Attitude to illness

Patients may consent to resuscitation procedures, but may be less at ease with long-term life-support procedures.

Blood transfusions

There are no objections to blood transfusions.

Contraception

- Most Orthodox Christians practise contraception, although the Church does not formally support it.
- Abortion is not generally accepted, except in emergencies.

Fertility treatment

In general this would be supported, but it is important to pay attention to each patient's particular circumstances.

Visiting

- Orthodox Christians emphasise the support that family life provides. At times of illness, members of the family will expect to be summoned to visit the patient.
- The patient may also request a visit from an Orthodox priest.

Dying and death

- The patient or a member of their family may request a priest to administer the sacraments (e.g. anointing, Holy Communion).

- Patients may wish to make their Confession, for which privacy will be needed.
- In areas where there are large Orthodox communities, a priest will be readily available. In smaller communities it is advisable to make plans in advance.
- Traditional practice is for the body to be buried, in keeping with a wish to maintain the integrity of the body after death.

Post-mortem

There are no objections to post-mortems.

Organ and tissue donation

- Organ and tissue donation is permitted, as the Orthodox Church teaches that such donation is an act of Christian love.
- Some people emphasise the importance of maintaining the physical integrity of the body after death, and therefore will not consent to organ or tissue donation.

Plymouth Brethren

This church is very strict in its social and religious code, prohibiting Brethren from mixing with non-Brethren people. The rationale is that they will eat and drink, and mix, only with those with whom they 'break bread' within the context of church worship. Such practice will inform their hospital experience and their choices.

- Patients may prefer the bed curtains to be closed while they are eating meals, in order to maintain strict privacy.
- Women do not cut their hair and they keep it covered in public, and during hospital admission.
- Men keep their hair short and are clean-shaven.
- There are no specific dietary requirements on religious grounds.
- At and after death the patient's relatives must be informed.
- A vigil may be kept at the bedside.
- After the patient's death the family will prefer to have complete control over what happens to the body, attending to the last offices and the washing of the body themselves.
- Unless required by law, post-mortems are not supported.
- Brethren object to heart transplants, believing the heart to be the seat of the affections.
- Kidney transplants are acceptable.
- No other transplants/organ donations are acceptable.

The Religious Society of Friends (Quakers)

- A Friend will usually receive pastoral-spiritual care provided by the local Meeting.
- There are no special dietary requirements on religious grounds.
- A Friend may wish the Clerk of the Meeting to know that they are dying, if they require spiritual support.
- There are no religious objections to post-mortem or to organ or tissue donation.

Seventh-Day Adventist Church

- Saturday is observed as the Sabbath, beginning on Friday at sunset.
- Members of this church may not eat pork, pork products or shellfish, in a pattern similar to the Jewish restrictions concerning kosher meat and fish.
- There are no specific religious requirements at the time of or after death. However, patients may welcome prayers, scripture readings and some sacramental ministry, and their local pastor should be contacted if necessary.
- Burial is normally preferred to cremation.
- There may be objections to post-mortem and to organ or tissue donation on religious grounds.

Other groups

Christian Science

Background and beliefs

Christian Science, established by Mary Baker Eddy, is a system of understanding and applying spiritual ideas to all aspects of life, including the healing or cure of disease. Christian Science is fully explained in Eddy's primary work, *Science and Health with Key to the Scriptures.* This healing system has been practised around the world for over a century by individuals of various faith traditions, as well as by those with no formal faith tradition. Some individuals choose to become members of the Church of Christ, Scientist, a church established by Mary Baker Eddy to make Christian Science healing more widely known and accessible.

Central to the practice of Christian Science is respect for individual choice in matters of healthcare or any other aspect of daily life. Many Christian Scientists rely on prayer for healing of diseases and disorders. However, individuals are free to choose conventional medical treatment.

Names

Christian Science is practised worldwide, and therefore naming will reflect ethnic diversity.

Religious obligations

- Christian Scientists may observe the main Christian festivals (e.g. Christmas, Easter).
- Patients may wish to engage in private prayer, and will welcome privacy for this.

Diet

Individuals make their own decisions about diet.

Dress

This may vary depending upon the patient's country of origin.

Language

Christian Scientists will reflect the diversity of their countries of origin in their language.

Birth

In keeping with their beliefs, women will prefer to give birth with as little medical intervention as possible, unless their safety and that of their baby is at risk.

Personal hygiene

Patients will need to maintain their own high standards of cleanliness. There are no religious requirements associated with this.

Gender, privacy and dignity

- Patients will appreciate being given privacy for their prayers.
- Christian Science patients will welcome an understanding response to their wish to be treated in specific ways in accordance with their belief system.

Attitude to illness

- In general, Christian Scientists avoid hospital treatment except in the case of childbirth or in the event of an accident.
- Christian Science patients may request that drugs/therapy be kept to a minimum, as they do not believe in medical interventions.
- If hospitalised due to an accident, Christian Scientists may decline conventional medical treatment.
- Patients may request re-testing or re-evaluation prior to an impending procedure after they have had time to pray for healing.
- Patients may ask if they can contact a Christian Science practitioner – that is, a professional spiritual healer who employs the Christian Science method of healing.

Blood transfusions

Individuals make their own decisions regarding blood transfusions, although transfusions are not generally regarded as acceptable. In the case of paediatric patients some parents may agree to a blood transfusion taking place.

Contraception

Individuals make their own decisions regarding contraception.

Fertility treatment

Christian Scientists do not endorse any intervention to assist or limit conception.

Visiting

- Patients will welcome a visit from a Christian Science practitioner in order to receive prayer for healing.
- A worldwide directory of Christian Science practitioners is available in *The Christian Science Journal*, a monthly periodical.

Dying and death

- There are no specified last rites. Such matters remain an individual or family decision.
- Whenever possible the body of a female patient should be prepared by a female member of healthcare staff.

Post-mortem

Christian Scientists will not generally support a post-mortem unless there is a legal requirement for it. However, it is essential that relatives are asked about this rather than erroneous assumptions being made.

Organ and tissue donation

Individuals or their relatives make their own decisions regarding organ or tissue donation.

Jehovah's Witness

Background and beliefs

During the late nineteenth century, the American Charles Taze Russell, who had become disaffected with traditional Christianity within his own denomination, established a new movement, which in 1931 became known as Jehovah's Witnesses. This is a religion whose members accept the Christian Bible as the word of God and endeavour to live by the laws and principles as contained within it.

Jehovah's Witnesses consider their religion to be in line with early Christianity. They accept the Old and New Testaments of the Bible, although they do not keep the traditional festivals of the church. Witnesses do not believe that Jesus Christ is equal with God, the Father (whom they refer to as Jehovah), and they do not believe in the traditional Christian doctrine of the Holy Trinity. One holy day is kept – the death of Christ – the date of which varies as it is calculated according to Biblical formula. Witnesses believe that Christ was crucified on a stake, not a cross, as they consider the latter to be pagan. Although they remember Christ's death, they do not celebrate Easter or Christmas. They believe in Satan, considering him to be God's enemy and the cause of many of the world's problems. Witnesses do not become involved in military service or in politics, nor do they celebrate birthdays. They show a deep commitment to their faith, a major element of which is the sharing of it (witnessing) with others. A key belief of the Witnesses is in Armageddon – the holy war between Christ and Satan, during which the world will be destroyed. Because of the rather frequent occasions on which Witnesses have foretold Armageddon, they are often mocked and criticised for their beliefs and lifestyle.

One of the fundamental beliefs of Jehovah's Witnesses is that taking blood into one's body is morally wrong. Patients will not accept treatment involving the use of blood or blood products, but will accept the use of non-blood-based medical management. Because of the religious and moral prohibition on the use of blood in healthcare, the children of Jehovah's Witnesses fall within the remit of the 1989 Children's Act. Jehovah's Witnesses believe that medical treatment is a matter for the informed consent of the individual.

Hospital Liaison Committees

The governing body of the Jehovah's Witnesses has created an international network of Hospital Liaison Committees in order to clarify their particular medical needs, and to gain support from medical staff in the use of bloodless procedures. Membership of the Liaison Committees consists of elders who have been specially trained to provide advice and information for doctors in relation to the provision of alternatives to blood products.

Names

As Jehovah's Witnesses are culturally diverse, their naming systems will vary.

Religious obligations

The only festival which is kept is that of the death of Christ, the date of which varies from one calendar year to the next.

Diet

- Because of the constraints upon the use of blood on religious grounds, some Witnesses are vegetarian.
- Witnesses who are not vegetarian will not wish to eat meat that contains blood or blood products, or meat from an animal that has been strangled, shot or not bled properly.

Dress

There are no specific issues concerning dress.

Language

This will be dependent upon the cultural/ethnic membership in a particular area.

Birth

There are no specific religious or pastoral requirements relating to birth, except in medical emergencies when the life of the mother and/or baby is at risk.

Personal hygiene

There are no specific religious requirements relating to personal hygiene.

Gender, privacy and dignity

- Witnesses are encouraged to 'keep Jehovah's organisation clean'. One of the ways in which this takes place is by members reporting the indiscretions of others to those in positions of authority.
- It is crucial that each patient is asked privately what information may be passed on to relatives.
- If a patient consents to the use of 'forbidden' blood products, there could be serious social consequences for them if this information became known.
- Healthcare staff should take extra care when discussing a Witness patient, in order to maintain privacy and confidentiality.

- Most Witnesses carry a special card identifying them as a Jehovah's Witness and releasing the hospital from responsibility in relation to the consequences of any limited treatment.

Attitude to illness

- Baptised Jehovah's Witnesses usually carry on their person an *Advance Directive/Release* document instructing that no blood transfusions should be given under any circumstances, and releasing doctors and hospitals from responsibility for any harm that might be caused by these patients' refusal of blood. This document is renewed annually.
- Many Witnesses also complete a more detailed *Healthcare Advance Directive* form that outlines their personal treatment choices with regard to blood 'fractions' and autologous blood procedures. A copy of this form is lodged with the patient's GP.
- When Witnesses are admitted to hospital, *Release Forms* should be signed which state matters similarly and deal more specifically with the hospital care and medical alternatives to blood transfusion that will be necessary.
- Sometimes these documents can be rescinded only in writing. Difficulties may arise if a patient is well enough to rescind the decision verbally, but not in writing.

Blood transfusions

- Jehovah's Witnesses believe that allogeneic blood transfusion is prohibited by Biblical passages in both the Old and New Testaments, and are therefore opposed to taking blood or blood products on these grounds. Blood is believed to be 'the soul of the flesh' ('But you must not eat the flesh with the life, which is blood, still in it,' Genesis 9.4). In the book of Leviticus it is stated that 'The life of every living creature is the blood, and I have forbidden the Israelites to eat the blood of any creature, because the life of every creature is its blood.' In the New Testament, the Acts of the Apostles states that 'You are to abstain from meat that has been offered to idols, from blood, from anything that has been strangled.'
- Witnesses refuse all blood transfusions, including stored autologous blood.
- Witnesses refuse red cells, white cells, plasma and platelets. However, they may elect to receive fractions of these components – for example, albumin, clotting factors, immunoglobins, interferon and haemoglobin-based oxygen carriers.
- The use of the blood patch technique as a haemostatic agent is a matter of personal choice.

- Many Witnesses will accept procedures such as intra-operative blood salvage and post-operative blood salvage from drains, as well as haemodilution techniques. To make such procedures acceptable, tubing should be visible to show that the diverted blood is still in contact with the patient, as tubing is regarded as an extension of the circulatory system.
- Witnesses are able to make their own decisions in some cases – for example, in relation to bone-marrow transplants, albumin, immuno-globulin and clotting factors.
- Witnesses expect blood to be handled with respect and neither stored nor reused.
- Some Witnesses may accept dialysis if they are reassured that only their blood is being used and that the extracorporeal circulation is continuous with the body circulation.
- Any changes in blood-product policy are conveyed to Witnesses through the *Watchtower* magazine.
- The Associated Jehovah's Witnesses for Reform on Blood has been established to reform and clarify the position of the religion as a whole with regard to the use of blood and blood products.

Contraception

Married couples privately and responsibly determine whether they will use appropriate methods of family planning. Witnesses avoid methods of contraception that induce abortion.

Fertility treatment

Attitudes to this may vary depending upon the type of treatment that is being proposed. Guiding principles will be the avoidance of unnecessary termination of a pregnancy and of the use of blood or blood products in any treatments.

Visiting

Jehovah's Witnesses have arrangements covering all of the main hospitals in the UK to provide spiritual support and practical assistance to Witness patients during periods of hospital admission.

Dying and death

- Jehovah's Witnesses have no special rituals or practices to perform for those who are dying, nor do they have specific last rites to be administered to those *in extremis.* Patients who are terminally ill will appreciate pastoral visits from elders.

- Jehovah's Witnesses will appreciate a quiet place for prayer with the patient and relatives.
- There is no religious objection to either burial or cremation.
- There are no special requirements to be observed by medical or nursing attendants at the time of death.

Post-mortem

There are no religious restrictions upon post-mortems.

Organ and tissue donation

- Witnesses may not wish to donate their organs on religious grounds, namely that another person's blood would flow through them. This prohibition is suspended in relation to the donation of corneas, which would not involve a flow of blood.
- Witnesses do support organ transplantation, although surgery of this kind would need to be performed in line with the guidelines for bloodless procedures.

Mormon (Church of Jesus Christ of Latter-Day Saints)

Background and beliefs

- The Church of Jesus Christ of Latter-day Saints was established in America in the early nineteenth century. The Old and New Testaments of the Bible are essential scriptures, along with the Book of Mormon.
- The Church views the Holy Trinity (Father, Son and Holy Spirit) as three separate and distinct members of a united Godhead.
- There is a belief in pre-existence – that is, a spirit life prior to birth. Life on earth is a period during which one has to prove that one is worthy to return to live in the presence of Jesus Christ and God the Father. Death is therefore understood as a temporary separation from loved ones.
- Family unity is of great importance. Family members who have died but who were not Mormons may be baptised into the faith and sealed to their families, so that they may be restored together after the resurrection.
- There is a strong emphasis on healthy living and the care of the body.

Names

There may be some cultural variations in the use of names, but most Mormons will follow the western form of naming.

Religious obligations

Members of the church who have undergone a special temple ceremony known as the *Endowment* wear sacred undergarments. These private garments are worn at all times. They may be removed in an emergency, but must be treated with respect. Members may choose not to wear these garments while they are inpatients.

Diet

- Mormons will not consume tea, coffee or alcohol, or use tobacco or other stimulants. Hot chocolate and other chocolate drinks are acceptable.
- Members may be vegetarian or choose to eat meat sparingly.

Gender, privacy and dignity

Members of the church who wear the sacred undergarment will appreciate sensitive awareness of this among healthcare staff.

Blood transfusions

There are no religious obligations with regard to blood transfusions.

Contraception

This is a matter for the individual couple, who will usually seek guidance from the scriptures and through prayer.

Dying and death

- Members of the church will expect to receive pastoral visits from representatives of the local congregation.
- Anointing with oil is common practice, with the intention of assisting in the healing of the sick person, along with the laying on of hands for healing. Patients will welcome privacy within the ward when this service takes place.
- The Sacrament (bread and water) is also brought to patients in hospital, although this is not standard practice.
- There are no specific last rites at the time of or after death. After death the deceased should be washed and dressed in a shroud.
- If the sacred garment has been worn, it must be replaced on the body after the deceased has been washed.
- Burial is preferred to cremation.

- The bishop of the church will provide pastoral support and assist with the funeral arrangements.
- The Relief Society will also assist with the practical arrangements for the funeral.
- The Church of Jesus Christ of Latter-Day Saints believes that a living being consists of two elements, namely the physical body and the spiritual body. Death causes the separation of the two elements. The spiritual body is eternal. After death, the physical body is destroyed, while the spiritual body waits for the day of resurrection.

Post-mortem

There are no religious objections to post-mortems.

Organ and tissue donation

There are no religious objections to organ and tissue donation. Family members are counselled and the decision is made by individuals and their families after competent medical advice has been given and confirmation received through prayer.

Rastafarian

Background and beliefs

- The Rastafarian movement originated in the 1920s in Jamaica, inspired by the teachings of a Jamaican, Marcus Garvey, who worked to promote the interests of people of African descent. The movement is linked to the roots of resistance to slavery among descendants of the black African slave families, and central to it is a strong bond with Africa. As the practice of Rastafarianism can vary widely, it is difficult to provide a clear definition.
- The essential belief of Rastafarians is that Haile Selassie I is the living God of the black race. The name was taken from the now dead Emperor of Ethiopia, Selassie, known as Ras Tafari – the Lion of Judah. Ras Tafari is believed to be the new Messiah, who will lead all black people to freedom.
- The Rastafarian name for God is Jah. The Lion of Judah represents Haile Selassie, the Conqueror. It also represents the King of Kings, as the lion is the king of beasts. Rastafarians do not regard themselves as Christians, as Christ was reborn in the new Messiah – Ras Tafari. However, they accept the Old and New Testament scriptures.
- Africa, and especially Ethiopia, is considered to be the Rastafarian's heaven on earth. There is no afterlife, in contrast to Christian belief.

Rastafarians believe that Jah will send the signal for the exodus back to Ethiopia, the Promised Land.

- There are sizeable Rastafarian communities in London, Leeds, Manchester, Birmingham, Liverpool, Bristol and Nottingham.
- The main aim of the movement is to bring about fundamental transformation of an unjust society.

Names

Some Rastafarians have biblical or Ethiopian names. Old Testament names (e.g. Moses, Zephaniah) are common.

Religious obligations

- Rastafarians follow the moral principles of the Ten Commandments, but follow the ancient laws of Ethiopia.
- Many Rastafarians belong to an organisation known as the Twelve Tribes of Israel. Its philosophy is to educate the young and assist the advancement of black people and the promotion of African and Ethiopian culture.
- The Rastafarian 'Livity' (way of life) is concerned with obeying Jah and recognising Ethiopia as the New Jerusalem and a spiritual homeland.
- Most Rastafarians do not belong to a church, although many of their beliefs are linked both to Christianity and to Judaism, because Rastafarianism is understood to be highly personal.
- Rastafarians will often use the Bible for guidance. In general their belief system is not rigid.
- Emphasis is given to mysticism, within a strong framework of personal spirituality. Meetings are held to discuss issues of importance and to provide support for members.
- Believers may be associated with the Ethiopian Orthodox or Judah Coptic churches.

Diet

- Many Rastafarians adhere to a system of dietary and hygiene laws that uphold and advocate a holistic lifestyle.
- Natural food that is as fresh and pure as possible is highly valued.
- Pork, predatory fish and some types of crustaceans are regarded as particularly unwholesome.
- Dairy products and refined and processed foods are avoided.
- Alcohol is rarely taken.
- Strict Rastafarians may be vegan.
- Some Rastafarians may wish to fast.

Dress

- Many Rastafarians wear their hair long and uncut in obedience to God. The dreadlocks and beard on men are regarded as a symbol of physical and moral strength and also of black pride.
- Dreadlocks symbolise the Rastafarian's roots, as well as representing the symbol of the Lion of Judah. Rastafarian women keep their heads covered during worship and when out in public places or receiving visitors.
- Some Rastafarians keep their heads covered at all times (with hairnets or scarves for women, and knitted woollen hats for men). Many Rastafarians may not agree to have their hair cut or shaved. If this is necessary it should be kept to a minimum.
- Modesty in dress is important. African influences may be seen in the fabrics and style of clothes worn.
- Hospital gowns that preserve dignity should be provided.
- Do not assume that someone is a Rastafarian on the basis of their appearance. Listen to the individual patient, as it is the individual who will inform healthcare practice.

Language

English is spoken by many Rastafarians.

Birth

- Rastafarian women will wish to give birth without excessive use of medical support, except in cases where the health of the baby or the mother is at risk.
- Breastfeeding is strongly encouraged. If bottle-feeding is necessary, women will wish to know the content of the milk and will avoid brands containing animal products.
- Circumcision is a matter of family choice.

Personal hygiene

Rastafarian patients maintain a high standard of personal cleanliness, and will wish to adhere to this in hospital.

Gender, privacy and dignity

- Hospital gowns are considered to be immodest, so the provision of more adequate covering will be appreciated.
- Women may wish to keep themselves covered at all times.
- Most female patients who require an internal examination will prefer this to be done by a female member of healthcare staff.

Attitude to illness

- The Rastafarian belief in the body's ability to heal itself may mean that a patient may be sceptical about invasive forms of medical treatment that 'interfere with God's plans.'
- Sensitivity to the patient's beliefs is important. Detailed information about the proposed treatment and all of the options available must be provided and discussed fully with the patient and their family.
- Some Rastafarians may use herbal remedies in conjunction with standard medication. Always check this in order to avoid adverse or impaired reactions to prescribed medication.

Blood transfusions

Blood transfusions may not be acceptable, so it is essential to check this with the patient or their relatives.

Contraception

Contraception is a matter of personal choice, although natural methods may be more acceptable.

Fertility treatment

Rastafarians highly value women's natural (unassisted) fertility. If a woman has difficulty in conceiving, she may therefore find it difficult to come to terms with any interventionist support.

Visiting

Rastafarians have a duty to visit the sick, and may do so in groups.

Dying and death

- Friends and relatives will visit and pray for a dying person.
- Sensitivity is required in order to provide appropriate spiritual care. As there is no formal structure within their organisation, an elder may approach staff with a request for the administration of last rites for the dying person.
- Some Rastafarians may wish to avoid touching a dead person, as to do so would necessitate shaving off their hair.
- There are no specific religious requirements at the time of or after death, so the body may be prepared in the usual way.
- Burial is preferred to cremation.

Post-mortem

In general a post-mortem is unacceptable unless there is a legal requirement for it. However, there may be exceptions to the general rule, and
healthcare staff should always check with the relatives.

Organ and tissue donation

Although there are no definitive guidelines, relatives may wish to confer
with the wider Rastafarian community before a decision is reached
concerning organ donation and transplant.

Hindu

Background and beliefs

Hinduism is a pluralistic religion which suggests that God can be thought of and approached in a variety of ways. This teaching is central to Hinduism. It emphasises that because we are all different, the ways in which we think of and approach the ultimate reality (i.e. God) will be different.

Hinduism offers a vast variety of concepts of God. These may be divided into three categories, namely God with form and quality, God without form, and God beyond the form and the formless. Hinduism does not advocate that any one approach is better than another. The choice is a matter for the individual.

The sanctity of life is central to Hindu teaching – Ahimsa. It teaches respect for living things, including the whole of the plant and animal kingdoms.

Hindus call Hinduism 'sanata dharma' – the eternal truth or religion. Its truth is believed to have been divinely revealed, and is passed down through the ancient scriptures known as the Veda.

Hinduism does not have a single founder, holy book or authority. There is immense diversity of belief and practice within Hinduism, depending upon an individual's country of origin and their family. Emphasis is given to the individual's beliefs and obligations.

Dharma is the name given to religious pursuits. It can mean righteous living, and it may be compared to the 'cohesive force that holds society and civilisation together.'

Hindu belief emphasises that all living beings possess a soul which passes through successive cycles of birth and rebirth. Hinduism, like Buddhism, includes the idea of karma and rebirth. Each person is believed to be reborn so that the soul may be purified and eventually join the cosmic consciousness. There are important emphases placed upon collective versus individual identity, and upon purity.

Hindus believe that a person does not live in isolation from their family, social group (caste) or environment.

Traditions that apply to all Asian cultures

- Shaking hands, hugging or embracing between the sexes is avoided when meeting members of the public, but is common between members of the same sex.
- Direct eye contact should be avoided when speaking to the patient, because it is regarded as a sign of disrespect.

- Try to maintain a formal approach during conversations.
- When meeting with a couple, direct the conversation towards the male partner only, or continue speaking to whoever takes the lead in the discussion.
- When talking with a couple, avoid referring to the wife as a 'partner.'
- Do not ask for a 'Christian name' when you mean the personal name of the patient.
- In matters of diagnosis, treatment and consent, the senior elder, and sometimes the extended family, will expect to be involved.
- A female patient may be reluctant to sign a consent form without first consulting her husband or father.

Names

- Hindu patients are likely to have three or four names – a given or personal name, a complimentary name (the father's name or the name of a deity), and a family name or surname.
- Use the surname or family name in all patient information, together with the personal name.
- Women who marry add their husband's first name and surname or family name to their personal name.
- The word 'bhai' (brother) may be added to men's personal names when used alone.
- The words 'bhai' or 'ben' may be added to women's names.

Religious obligations

- The individual is free to worship God in many and varied ways, and may choose to worship those deities with whom he or she feels a particular affinity.
- There are no set times for prayers.
- Puja/worship may take place in a temple in front of the deities, or at home.
- Prayers can be said individually, with the family, or in a large gathering.
- A devout Hindu may say prayers (do Puja) in the morning after a shower, in the evening, and before going to bed.
- In the UK, Hindus usually gather for worship on Saturday and Sunday.
- Festivals take place throughout the year, the most important one being Diwali. This is a festival of lights that takes place in October or November.

Diet

- The different regions of India each have their own dietary practices.
- Reverence for life ('Ahimsa' – mental, physical and emotional non-injury of all beings) is central to dietary practice.

- Check the dietary requirements of each individual Hindu patient.
- Some Hindus will be vegetarian.
- Most Hindus do not eat beef or pork. The cow is a sacred animal and the pig is seen as a scavenging animal whose meat is dirty.
- Some Hindus will eat eggs.
- Dairy produce is acceptable so long as it does not contain animal fat.
- Strict vegetarian Hindus will not eat off a plate or with the same utensils that have been used to serve meat. Plastic plates and cutlery should be supplied in these circumstances.
- Certain foods are classified as 'hot' or 'cold' in terms of their effect both on the body and on the emotions. Hot foods are salty, sour or high in animal protein. It is thought that they increase the body temperature and excite the emotions. Cold foods are generally sweet or bitter and are thought to lower the body temperature, calm the emotions and help the person to be strong and happy. It is believed that dietary imbalances create physical and emotional ill health.
- There are no set rules for fasting. The decision to fast is taken individually, and may also include abstaining from speaking.
- When fasting does take place, cooked foods will not be eaten but a drink may be taken. Check with the individual concerned.
- Hindu people prefer to eat using their right hand only.

Dress

- Most Punjabi women (Muslim, Sikh or Hindu) wear Shalwar-Kamees. Shalwar are baggy trousers that have narrowed ankles and are tied around the waist using a waist lace. Kamees is a long top or shirt.
- It is common for Hindu men to wear western clothing.
- Girls often wear traditional clothes at home and western clothing outside the home.
- Asian women wear the Dupatta or Chunni, consisting of two and a half yards of material draped around the top half of the body in a variety of ways, sometimes covering the head.
- The sari is also the most common form of dress for women and is worn in many different ways, depending upon the region from which the patient originates.
- Hindu women consider the wearing of jewellery to be something sacred as well as sentimental. It is passed from one generation to the next.

Language

- Many Hindus speak English in addition to their own language.
- Hindus may speak Gujarati, Hindi, Punjabi and Bengali.
- Sanskrit is the language of Hindu sacred texts and is not a conversational language.

- When an interpreter is needed, efforts should be made to find one who is familiar with the patient's own traditions and culture. It is crucial that the interpreter can be relied upon to interpret accurately and without censorship.

Miscarriage, stillbirth and neonatal death

- If miscarriage takes place before the seventh month of pregnancy, no religious rites are required, although some parents may wish for some formal recognition of the birth and death of their baby.
- Stillborn babies are usually buried rather than cremated. This principle also applies in the case of neonatal death.
- A woman may suffer considerable guilt and shame if she has more than one pregnancy loss, whether due to miscarriage or stillbirth, as the Hindu emphasis is upon a woman's fertility and ability to bear children.

Birth

- The fetus is considered to be a person from the moment of conception, so abortion is unacceptable except in emergencies.
- Hindus believe in rebirth (i.e. that the soul is reborn many times in different bodies).
- During pregnancy the mother is encouraged to read the Hindu scriptures and to meditate. These practices are believed to encourage a positive birth into this life.
- Punsavana – the fetus ceremony – takes place during the third or fourth month of pregnancy to invoke divine qualities in the infant.
- The seventh month of pregnancy is significant, as it is believed to be the month when the soul enters the body. Further prayers – Simantonnayana – are said at this stage.
- If miscarriage takes place before the seventh month there are no religious requirements. If the baby dies from the seventh month of gestation onwards, a funeral should take place.
- After birth the baby is ceremonially washed and a golden pen dipped in honey is used to write the word AUM on his or her tongue. This ceremony may be delayed until the mother and child return home. Not all Hindus will have this ceremony performed.
- The naming ceremony takes place on the tenth day after birth. The priest draws up the baby's horoscope and chooses the first letter of his or her name.
- Mothers are traditionally expected to rest for 40 days after giving birth, in order to regain their strength.
- Gifts of clothes for the new baby are acceptable.
- The birth of a boy – the first boy – is especially welcome. There is a religious and cultural preference for sons.

Personal hygiene

- Purity (Suddha) is very important within Indian culture, creating the concept of the human body as pure, perfect and a desired state of being. Physical cleanliness is linked to Suddha and leads to the meticulous practice of personal hygiene.
- Most Hindus are accustomed to having water in the same room as the toilet.
- If there is no tap or bidet, or if a bedpan has to be used, then a container of water for washing should be provided.
- Hindu patients prefer to wash in free-flowing water (e.g. a shower or a bucket of water) rather than sit in a bath.
- Women are regarded as unclean during menstruation, and will take a special shower at the end of this time.
- Washing the hands before and after a meal is expected.
- Patients will also wish to rinse out their mouths after eating.

Gender, privacy and dignity

- Hindu women prefer to be seen by female healthcare staff.
- Long gowns should be provided for women who are being prepared for X-ray or surgery.
- Hindu women and men expect to be placed in single-sex wards to avoid embarrassment.

Attitude to illness

- Hindus believe that suffering has meaning.
- Illness is thought to be punishment for wrong behaviour in a former life.
- Sometimes blessed articles of jewellery will be placed on a black string on a patient's body. This is seen as a form of protection.
- Hindus maintain a positive attitude to illness, striving to maintain hope.
- In general, Hindu patients will accept the authority of medical staff, whether male or female.
- Hindus may prefer home remedies for illness, and consequently may be slow to seek medical advice.

Contraception

- There are no specific religious rules concerning contraception, although some traditions may offer particular guidance.
- Forms of contraception that might cause irregular periods or spotting may be inappropriate in view of the religious restrictions imposed upon menstruating women. However, it is important for medical practitioners to inform women in these circumstances that such bleeding does not fall within such religious constraints.

- In general, abortion is not supported. However, there are exceptions to this rule, especially when a woman's life is at risk.

Fertility treatment

This will be a matter for specific consideration with the couple involved. Given the emphasis upon a woman's natural fertility, and a general reluctance to terminate pregnancy, this matter may be a difficult concept for some Hindus.

Visiting

It is expected that the family will visit continually throughout a person's hospital admission. This may necessitate hospital staff considering an extension of visiting hours to meet these needs, especially at times of crisis.

Dying and death

- The patient may wish to die at home, as this has particular religious significance.
- It is important that all close family members are present. They may wish to pray at the bedside and to make sure that all religious rites take place.
- The family may wish to be actively involved in the care of the patient, and should be asked if this is their wish.
- The patient's eldest son is expected to be present before, during and after death. This pertains even when that son is a small child.
- Families who have not performed the essential rituals may become anxious about the spiritual consequences both for themselves and for the well-being of the soul of the dead patient.
- A Hindu patient or relative may request the services of a Hindu priest/ Pandit during the last stages of life to perform the following holy rites in order to assist with the transmigration of their soul at death:
  - tying a thread around the neck or wrist to bless the dying person
  - sprinkling water from the River Ganges over the person
  - placing the sacred Tulsi leaf in the mouth
  - if possible the patient may wish to be placed on the floor on a sheet or a mat, to symbolise closeness to Mother Earth, freedom from physical constraints, and the easing of the soul's departure.
- The patient may derive some comfort from the hymns and readings of the holy books. Some may wish for images or pictures, praying beads or blessings (flowers) on or near the bed.
- Some Hindus are strict about who may touch the body after death. For example, some may feel distressed if a non-Hindu touches the body.
- Close family members usually wash the body, and may request to do this on the ward. Traditionally the eldest son takes a leading role in the washing and dressing of the body.

- The eyes are closed and the legs straightened.
- The hair or beard must not be trimmed without the relatives' consent.
- Some Hindus may wish to light a clay lamp using a piece of cotton wool soaked in ghee. Others may wish to burn an incense stick in the room.
- The patient's relatives must be consulted before any of the medical staff handle the body.
- If the relatives consent to the body being touched by non-Hindus, the following conditions apply:
  - female patients should only be handled by female medical staff
  - male patients should only be handled by male medical staff.
- Jewellery, sacred threads and other religious objects should be left in place.
- The body should be covered with a plain white sheet.
- Close relatives will wish to pay their last respects while the body remains on the ward.
- The eldest son or another male relative will attend to the funeral arrangements.
- In India and elsewhere the body is cremated within 24 hours of death.
- The hospital should try to release the body as soon as possible so that the family may make arrangements for the cremation.
- Infants and young children under 5 years of age may be buried.
- The family will not cook food until the cremation/burial has taken place.

Post-mortem

- Post-mortems are generally regarded as unacceptable. However, there may be exceptions to this general rule dependent upon individual circumstances.
- Hindus will be anxious for the return of all organs to the body before cremation (or burial for a child under 5 years of age) in order to secure peace in the afterlife.

Organ and tissue donation

- There are many references in Hindu scriptures that support the concept of organ donation. *Daan* is the original word for donation in Sanskrit, meaning 'selfless giving.'
- Organ donation is an integral part of the Hindu way of life as guided by the Vedas.
- Scientific treatises form an important part of the Vedas. Sage Charaka deals with internal medicine, while Sage Sushruta includes features of organ and limb transplants.

Islam

Background and beliefs

The word 'Islam' means peace and submission, implying a peaceful way of life based on submission to the will of God/Allah. The Islamic faith is followed by many Muslims throughout the world, although there is considerable diversity of belief and thought within the faith.

A Muslim may be defined as a person who accepts the Islamic way of life, and who complies with the will of God without question.

Muslims believe that Mohammed is the prophet sent by God for all humanity. They believe that the holy book, Qur'an, is the revealed book of Allah. Mecca is the birthplace of the prophet Mohammed and is a place of profound significance for all Muslims. The Ka'bah (a cubical building built by the Prophet Abraham) is in Mecca, and it is in the direction of this building that Muslims turn for their prayers.

There are five fundamental principles that are to be practised by every Muslim.

1 Belief in the oneness of God. To bear witness that there is no one worthy of worship but Allah, and that Mohammed is Allah's servant and apostle for all humanity.
2 The reciting of five daily prayers (Salat) – in the early morning before sunrise, at noon, between noon and sunset, at sunset, and at night. These prayers are obligatory and can be offered anywhere. Friday afternoon prayer is the weekly congregational prayer.
3 Fasting during Ramadan from dawn to dusk. This involves one month of abstinence from food and drink. Ramadan occurs 11 days earlier each year, and is the ninth month of the Islamic calendar. Seriously ill people, menstruating, pregnant and breastfeeding women, elderly people in poor health, and children are exempt from the fast.
4 The giving of alms (Zakat).
5 Pilgrimage to Mecca once in a lifetime.

In the UK the majority of Muslims come from India and Pakistan. More recent settlers in the UK include Muslims from Turkey, Cyprus, Somalia, Bosnia, Ethiopia, Algeria and Morocco.

Names

Since Islam spans many countries and cultures there are names and name patterns that reflect both Islamic and local cultures. However, the following points must be remembered.

1 When Muslims marry, the woman does not usually change her name.
2 Children do not necessarily have their father's name.
3 A surname or family name may not necessarily exist.
4 People of all origins may add certain titles to names to show respect (e.g. Bibi and Begum for women). Men who are especially devout may have extra religious titles added.
5 The last name is not a shared family surname. In most Muslim families each member has a different name. For example:
   - husband: Mohammed Hafiz
   - wife: Jameela Khatoon
   - sons: Mohammed Sharif and Liaquat Ali
   - daughter: Fatima Jan.

This can cause difficulties for the following reasons.

- Most records are recorded under the husband's name, and it is this name which must be asked for, irrespective of which person (husband or wife) you are addressing.
- It cannot be assumed that, for example, Liaquat Ali's father is also called Ali.
- Some families who have settled in the UK have adopted a surname, but this may not appear on any official document (passport, etc.). The 'surname' used in UK records is often the husband's personal name.
- Female Muslims also have a two-part name, although neither part has religious significance.
- The first name is always a personal name, as in the British system.
- The second name can either be a title (e.g. Bano, Begum, Bibi, Khatoon, Sultana) or another personal name (e.g. Akhtar, Jan, Kausar).
- The second name should be used for the purposes of recording the patient's details formally. Because the husband's name is different, cross-referencing will be needed.

Religious obligations

To pray five times daily
Prayers may be conducted anywhere that is convenient and clean. During illness prayers may be said sitting up or lying down, so long as the chair or bed is facing Mecca. *In major illness patients are exempt from prayer.* If there is no prayer mat available, a folded sheet or a clean towel may be used instead. The patient may draw the curtains for privacy. As the prayers do not take long (10–15 minutes), this should not cause difficulties on the ward. Some Muslims wear a Ta'weez (amulet) around their neck. This is a religious article inscribed with Qur'anic verses as a protection against evil.

Cleansing

Cleansing (Wusu or Ghusal) must be performed before touching the Qur'an. It takes the form of handwashing, gargling, rinsing the mouth and nostrils, washing the face and the arms, passing wet hands over the hair, and washing the feet. A normal wash hand basin is adequate for performing the Ablution, but the patient may need assistance if they are elderly, frail or weak.

The direction of the Quibla

Muslims must face south-east towards the Quibla/Ka'bah in Mecca. A compass helps to find the direction for prayer. A Quibla sign may be put on the wall to avoid the need for constant use of a compass.

The Holy Qur'an

This is the most important holy book for Muslims. The Qur'an should be handled only after Ablution, and must be treated with care and respect.

Ramadan

This period of fasting usually falls in the latter part of each year, although the calendar dates will vary. Muslims are permitted to eat and drink before sunrise, but must then fast until dusk. Ramadan is a period of spiritual discipline. Children are taught to pray and keep the fast when they reach adolescence.

The sick and infirm and also menstruating women are not expected to fast during Ramadan. However, some patients may wish to keep the fast while in hospital. It is important to discuss the implications of fasting with the patient and/or their relatives in order to reach an agreement about this and for medical opinion to be taken seriously in cases where fasting would further damage the patient's health. During illness a person may be given a temporary or permanent exemption from the requirement to fast, especially when fasting would worsen the condition. Patients with chronic illness may be encouraged to engage in other disciplines, such as giving alms, rather than fasting.

Practical considerations include the following.

- Although the use of oral medicine is prohibited while fasting, it is possible to adjust the preparations and the dosage times so that medication may be taken outside the hours of fasting.
- Healthcare providers need to consider how the regular appointments system for patients might be adjusted to take into account the different eating, waking and sleeping patterns of most Muslims during Ramadan.
- Community practitioners (GPs, health visitors, nurses, etc.) would benefit from training in how to manage fasting patients in relation to medical care.

Eid

Eid-ul-fitr is celebrated immediately after Ramadan and is the festival of breaking the fast. This is the Muslim community's assertion of unity and family solidarity. It is a community and family celebration. Presents, new clothes and money are given to children.

Eid-ul-Adha is the festival commemorating the Prophet Abraham's willingness to sacrifice his son, Ismail, in obedience to God's command. This festival falls on the day after the day of Hajj.

Diet

- Lamb, beef, goat, chicken, rabbit, deer, etc. can be consumed provided that a Muslim has slaughtered these, after prayers have been said. This is Halal food.
- Pakistani Muslims are strict about eating only Halal meat.
- Pork meat, all pork products and blood are forbidden.
- Wine and other alcoholic drinks are also forbidden.
- Muslims do not eat meat or other food containing animal fats, or fats from animals which have not been ritually slaughtered.
- Fish and eggs are permitted. These must not be cooked in conjunction with pork or non-Halal meat.
- Patients may ask their relatives to bring Halal food from home, as this is more culturally appropriate.
- Some second-generation Muslims will eat English food (e.g. vegetables, fish, rice).
- In cooking, meat or meat products such as gelatine must be avoided.
- Separate utensils for cooking and serving the Halal food are essential.

Dress

- Muslims are required to follow rules of modesty in their dress, especially in public places where the two sexes meet.
- Women are required to cover their head (the Hijab) and to wear loose clothing.
- In some traditions women also cover their faces.
- Some men may wear a small cap, especially during prayer.
- As Muslims represent many Eastern and African cultures, there is a diversity of cultural dress among Muslims in the UK.

Language

- Depending upon their country of origin, Muslims will speak a variety of different languages.

- Some Muslims will speak English alongside the language of their country of origin.
- Languages spoken by Muslims include the following:
  - Punjabi, Urdu, Pushto and Bengali
  - Serbo-Croat
  - Amharic (Ethiopia)
  - Gujarati, Hausa and Malay
  - Somali, Arabic and Hamito-Semetic (Somalia)
  - Turkish and Kurdish.

Birth

Birth ceremonies include a number of elements.

- The Adhan is the Muslim call to prayer. After birth the baby is washed and the Adhan is called softly into its right ear. The Iqamat is said into the baby's left ear.
- Something sweet (a small piece of date or some honey) is placed in the baby's mouth soon after birth.
- The baby is named on the seventh day after birth.
- The baby's head is shaved on the seventh day after birth.
- All boys are circumcised.
- Islam does not sanction female circumcision.

Personal hygiene

- Islam emphasises the importance of cleanliness. Before any worship Muslims must ensure that their clothes are clean, and perform a cleansing ritual known as Ghusal or Wusu.
  - Ghusal is a complete body wash with clean water, and is performed after lovemaking and after menstruation.
  - Wusu is a partial wash with clean water, and is performed before prayer. Wusu is void after urination, defecation, passing wind or vomiting, and must be repeated.
- Muslims prefer to wash their genitals with running water after using the toilet. This is called Istinja. A jug provided for this purpose in the toilet or bathroom is appreciated.
- Muslims use their left hand for toileting and their right hand for eating, etc. This requirement must be remembered when choosing a hand for intravenous drugs. Staff must ask the patient which hand may be used.
- If a bedpan or commode is used, fresh water must be provided for cleansing.
- Although nurses and non-Muslims are allowed to wash sick people, social conventions may apply with regard to modesty, gender and body parts. It is important to ask the patient about this, as social and cultural conventions vary.

Gender, privacy and dignity

- Men are believed to be the protectors of women. It is therefore important that they are consulted about any treatment for their wives or sisters.
- Muslims take their membership of both family and the Muslim community very seriously. In some circumstances relatives may wish to consult community elders. In life-threatening circumstances, or when there is no immediate male member of the family available, a female relative may give consent.
- Muslims regard modesty in dress as extremely important.
- A man must cover his body from the navel to the knees.
- A woman is required to cover her whole body except for the feet and the hands.
- The clothing must not be tight or transparent, and must conceal the shape of the body.
- All medical gowns must respect this need for modesty (e.g. the gowns must be suitably long and completely cover the patient's body).
- Muslims prefer to be examined by medical staff of the same gender. When circumstances do not allow this, the rules can be waived. However, some Muslim women may wish a female relative or member of staff to be present during medical examinations that are conducted by a male member of the healthcare staff.
- Muslims prefer accommodation in single-sex wards or bays.
- Muslims would not usually expect to have medical information discussed directly with the patient, preferring to refer the matter to second-degree male relatives (e.g. uncles or cousins).

Attitude to illness

- Muslims believe that nothing can take place without the consent of Allah, according to his judgment and distinction, as nothing can happen against his will.
- Illness and suffering are regarded as a means of purification, and as a punishment for wrongdoing. A period of illness is understood as providing an opportunity to make peace with one's family and community, and with God.
- Muslims believe in a life after death, when the individual will be judged. Heaven and hell form part of the judgment given by God.
- In adversity a Muslim is forbidden to despair and is required to be patient, seeking help through prayers and remembrance of Allah.
- Islam emphasises the exercising of compassion and sympathy for the terminally ill.
- Muslims may not always display emotion during times of crisis brought about by illness, or at the death of a relative.

- Muslims may be reluctant to take drugs. During Ramadan a Muslim patient may wish to receive only essential medications.
- A Muslim woman may not wish to make important medical decisions without her husband or father present.

Blood transfusions

- In general, there are no Islamic objections to blood transfusions.
- There may be exceptions, so consultation with the patient and/or relatives is important.

Religious implications of menstruation

- Muslim women are exempt from regular prayers, fasting and undertaking the Hajj during menstruation. Although sexual intercourse is forbidden at this time, other forms of physical contact between husband and wife are permitted.
- Women may be reluctant to attend a gynaecological clinic on the basis that if an internal examination takes place this may cause bleeding. The same reason will apply to women's non-attendance at regular family planning clinics in relation to the use of the IUD.
- Many Muslim women will not realise that the religious requirements do not apply when bleeding has been induced as a result of medical examination.
- By contrast, some women will visit their GP in order to control the menstrual pattern, particularly in advance of the Pilgrimage to Mecca (Hajj). In such circumstances, oral contraceptives are provided.

Contraception

- There are varying attitudes to contraception within the Muslim community. In general the understanding is that although contraception is allowed, it is also discouraged. However, the personal autonomy of the couple is recognised, and in practice individuals will vary widely in their contraceptive practices.
- The proportion of Muslim women who use some form of contraception is lower than that among other ethnic communities.
- Any discussion must be held in confidence and discretely – never in front of visiting relatives or friends.
- The IUD appears to be the contraceptive method most favoured by Muslim women, despite the increased risks of bleeding. Possible reasons for this choice include the fact that it keeps any medical contact at a low level, including the need for consultations with a male doctor.
- Some Muslim women use oral contraceptives.

- Muslims are generally less likely to terminate pregnancies on the grounds of any abnormality. However, it must not be assumed that because Islam discourages abortion, Muslim parents should not be offered any opportunity to discuss the matter further. It is important to regard the religious framework as a crucial context in which to discuss all possibilities as fully as possible with the parents.
- Abortion is not permitted except in an emergency.
- Abortion is not permitted in cases of rape or incest, as Islam emphasises the right of the child to life.
- Permitted abortion must take place before 120 days (approximately 3 months), as according to Islam the soul is breathed into the fetus after this time. This is termed 'ensoulment.'

Fertility treatment

- Within Islam, the child's rights take precedence over those of the parents. Such rights commence even before conception, and are related to the choice of a marriage partner.
- Given this context, Islam does not support fertility treatment that uses donor sperms and eggs.
- The use of the husband's sperm in artificial insemination is generally accepted.

Miscarriage, stillbirth and neonatal death

- Not all Muslims would ascribe personhood to a fetus that is less than 24 weeks' gestation. Muslims regard the ability to breathe as indicative of life and of personhood.
- There is no religious recognition and ritual for the burial of a fetus at less than 24 weeks' gestation. However, some parents have requested the presence of a Mufti or an Imam immediately following a miscarriage.
- Fetal remains must be buried.
- Any baby that is stillborn must be given a name.
- The baby must be buried, although there is no formal religious ceremony.
- Some parents may wish photographs to be taken of the baby, although within Islam photographs or images of the human form are forbidden.

Visiting

- Visiting a sick relative or friend is a faith obligation and is regarded by Muslims as a virtuous act, which is greatly rewarded by God.
- A large number of people may visit a Muslim patient to pray with and for them.

- At times of crisis many people will wish to visit. It is important for ward staff to set certain guidelines for visiting, in order to respect the needs of other patients in the area, while supporting the wish of Muslims to visit the person who is ill.

Dying and death

- Muslims understand death to be a 'marker' of the transition from one state of being to another. Rather than fearing or fighting death, Muslims are encouraged to accept death as part of the will of Allah.
- Although Islam does not support suicide or euthanasia, equally it does not support undue suffering. There is a positive attitude to the use of pain relief.
- When a Muslim patient is near death, the relatives and/or a member of the local Mosque committee should be informed.
- In ideal circumstances Muslims much prefer to be able to die at home.
- If it is not possible for the patient to return home in order to die, generous provision must be made for relatives and friends to visit him or her. It is usual for many people to visit the dying person, and ward staff must try to make adequate space available. Visitors will sit by the patient's bed and recite verses from the Qur'an, and pray for the peaceful departure of the soul.
- The time before death is important for the extending of forgiveness among family and friends.
- The patient should be turned to face Mecca and the direction of the Ka'bah (Quibla). Turn the patient on their right side, facing south-east.
- If the patient is unable to be turned, they may be placed on their back with their feet facing in a south-east direction and their head raised slightly.
- If the patient is conscious, they will be encouraged to recite the Declaration of Faith.
- When the patient dies, the recitation of the Qur'an ceases immediately.
- Relatives will wish to:
  - close the eyes of the deceased
  - turn the body to the right, and if possible towards the Quibla
  - bandage the lower jaw to the head so that the mouth does not gape
  - flex the joints of the arms and legs to stop them becoming rigid, to enable washing and shrouding.
- A complete cleansing will take place (Ghusal). Relatives may wish to do this on the ward. Alternatively they may wait until the body is removed to their own undertakers.
- No hair or nails must be cut.
- The body will be wrapped in a Caffan. In the absence of a Caffan, a white sheet is acceptable.
- At all times the body must be covered with due regard to modesty.

- Nursing staff may fulfil the above requirements if no relatives or representatives are present. Use disposable gloves if necessary.
- The body must be released to the relatives or to the local Muslim community, who will make arrangements for the washing, shrouding and burial according to Islamic regulations.
- Any tubes, etc. or artificial limbs should be removed.
- Any incisions should be plugged to prevent or stem a flow of blood.
- Muslims do not usually bury the corpse in a coffin, but if the law or other special circumstances require it, they will not object to this.
- Burial must take place as quickly as possible.
- The relatives will be grateful for a speedy release of the body, legal requirements permitting.
- The body of a deceased woman must be handled only by female healthcare staff.
- The body of a deceased man must be handled only by male healthcare staff.
- If relatives or members of the Muslim community are not available to take charge of the body, it may be kept in the mortuary for a short time.

End of life/resuscitation

- Muslims believe that a person who has been pronounced medically brain-dead should not be kept alive artificially.
- Resuscitation is permitted, but only after careful consultation with the family. In certain circumstances resuscitation may take place for medical reasons.

Post-mortem

- The general opinion within Islam is that post-mortem examinations are not acceptable. One of the reasons given for this is that a post-mortem will delay the burial of the body. Another reason is that according to Islamic belief the deceased may still be able to feel or perceive pain. In general the desecration of the body in this way is not supported.
- Where it is essential, for legal reasons, for a post-mortem to take place, it is crucial that the relatives are fully consulted.
- In circumstances where it is intended that a post-mortem examination will be performed for educational purposes, full consultation with the family is essential.

Organ and tissue donation

- In 1996 the Muslim Law Council (UK) issued a fatwa (religious opinion) on organ donation.

- The council supports organ transplantation as a means of alleviating pain or saving life on the basis of the rules of the Shariah.
- Muslims may carry donor cards.
- The next of kin of a dead person, in the absence of a card or an expressed wish to donate their organs, may give permission to obtain organs from the body in order to save other people's lives.
- The fatwa is based on the Islamic principle of 'necessities overruling prohibition.' Violation of the human body is usually forbidden in Islam, but the Shariah believes that this can be overruled when saving another person's life.
- However, there are also a significant number of Muslim scholars who believe that organ donation is not permissible, and who hold the view that this does not fall within the criteria of 'necessity overruling prohibition', due to other overriding Islamic principles.
- Both viewpoints take their evidence from the Qur'an and the Ahaadith.
- Individual Muslims should make a decision according to their understanding of the Shariah or seek advice from the local Imam or Mufti/scholar.

Jain

Background and beliefs

Jains do not believe in a supreme creator God, but rather they believe that the universe has always existed. They revere and worship the 24 teachers (conquerors or pathfinders) of their faith. Mahavira, who was a contemporary of the Buddha, was the last and most recent teacher, in the sixth century BC, who revived and reformulated Jainism, and is especially honoured.

The principle of Karma, which Jains teach, is that the body inhabited by a soul in its next life is determined mainly by the soul's present actions. The human state is the only one from which release from the cycle of birth and death is possible. The teachings of the Tirthankaras lead humans to spiritual release.

Ascetism, prayer and practice enable the five Jain ideals of human development. Although there are several levels of spiritual development, most Jains are lay people whose lifestyles are influenced by the Five Great Vows of Jain Monastics. Jains believe that all souls have characteristics of infinite perception, knowledge, energy and bliss. However, these capacities of the self are restricted by karma, which is responsible for perverted conduct, injustices, rebirth and transmigration. The meaning of life is to shed karma by self-effort and free the soul from its bondage so that it can live at the apex of the universe, from where there is no rebirth.

Jainism believes in the equality of all souls, irrespective of caste, belief, race or culture, and in reverence for life as a whole. Jains are encouraged to adhere to the following key principles:

- non-violence and compassion for all living creatures
- truthfulness
- not stealing
- celibacy and chastity
- non-attachment and non-ownership
- multiplicity of views.

There is a graduated pathway known as the Three Jewels that leads towards release from karma. This pathway, which is followed by both lay people and monks and nuns, consists of the following:

- right faith
- right knowledge
- right conduct.

Since Jains and Hindus have lived side by side for thousands of years, they share some common traditions and practices.

Names

A Jain patient is likely to have three names:

- a personal first name
- a complimentary middle name
- a family surname.

The family surname should be used on the medical records. In general it is polite to use the patient's title plus their surname, especially when addressing an elderly person.

Religious obligations

- Prayer and worship. Jains may worship at home shrines three times a day – before dawn, at sunset and at night. They may also worship at temples, or will meet in homes or in halls.
- Fasting (tapas – practices of austerity). This may involve fasting from one meal a day, or fasting for an entire day or longer.

Diet

- Jains may eat milk, curd and ghee.
- Prohibited foods include meat, fish, eggs, butter, root vegetables, figs, honey and alcohol. Some Jains may also abstain from eating garlic and onions.
- Strict Jains may not eat after sunset or before sunrise.
- When preparing or storing food, keep prohibited foods separate from Jain foods.
- Some Jains may prefer to eat with the curtains closed in order to avoid seeing other patients eating meat, etc.
- It is a good idea to ask Jain patients whether an Asian vegetarian diet is acceptable to them, or if they require special food.
- Relatives are often willing to bring in food, so long as facilities are available for storage and heating the food.
- When fasting, Jains will not take anything except boiled water during the day. Fasting may take place on the fifth and/or fourteenth day of each lunar month. Jains may also fast for a week during the festival of Paryusana-parva in August or September.

Dress

Many Jains will wear Asian clothing, maintaining physical modesty.

Language

Jains may speak Hindi and/or Urdu, as well as English. An interpreter may be required for older patients.

Birth

It is customary for a Jain woman to rest for 40 days after giving birth, although Jain patients will adapt to the rules of the hospital. The relatives assist the mother in regaining her strength following the birth, and in caring for the baby.

Personal hygiene

Some Jains may prefer water for washing after using the toilet. There are no other specific requirements.

Gender, privacy and dignity

Female patients will usually prefer a female doctor and nurse to attend them.

Attitude to illness

- Some Jains may choose to avoid certain drugs, the taking of which may break the commitment against harming any form of life (e.g. antibiotics).
- Some Jains may also be reluctant to take opiates, due to their emphasis upon endurance, self-discipline and suffering.
- Although Jain patients may rely on spiritual practices and on human support and comfort, nevertheless they will also co-operate both with medical staff and in their own medical care.

Blood transfusions

There are no objections to blood transfusions.

Contraception

There are no religious obligations placed upon Jains with regard to contraception. However, they will avoid abortion if contraception fails. It is advisable to discuss the use of the most reliable form of contraception with couples.

Visiting

Jain patients will welcome visits both by members of their family and by other members of their religious community. A visit by the Brahman is especially welcome.

Dying and death

- A Jain patient who is seriously ill may derive comfort from meditation, the worship of holy images, prayer beads, prayer books, and recordings of mantras and prayers.
- Jains believe that the individual should have good thoughts, with a feeling of detachment as death approaches. The prayers and other devotions are aids to this detachment.
- It is very important that the patient's family is present. This may present difficulties both with regard to space in a ward or a side room, and in relation to the needs of other patients.
- The relatives may wish to chant or to pray with the patient.
- The relatives may chant in the patient's ear, even if he or she is not conscious.
- Some Jains may wish to burn incense, in which case careful explanation of the fire safety regulations will be advisable.
- Jain patients may wish to ask for forgiveness from relatives and friends if they have harmed them either knowingly or unknowingly. Repentance, confession and penance are very strong beliefs for Jains in relation to karma.
- The patient may wish to make a donation to a charitable cause.
- When a Jain patient is elderly or very ill, or no further treatment is appropriate for them, they may choose to withdraw from the world by means of fasting. This is in order to undertake a 'holy death.' The patient may then fast for lengthy periods, reducing their food intake until only fluids are taken, and finally reducing their fluid intake. They may also refuse all medication in such circumstances.

Post-mortem

Post-mortem is regarded as being disrespectful to the body. However, this attitude will vary depending upon the orthodoxy of the individual's beliefs.

Organ and tissue donation

There is generally no objection to organ donation and transplants. However, it is good practice to check this information with the individual and/or their immediate relatives or next of kin.

Jewish

Background and beliefs

Judaism is based on the belief in one universal God, seen by Jews in a personal relationship. The love of God and the wish to carry out the Ten Commandments as given to Moses on Mount Sinai are embodied in the teaching of the Pentateuch (the first five books of the Old Testament).

The three elements of Judaism are as follows.

1 **God.** God exists. God is one. God is not in bodily form. God is eternal. God knows the deeds of human beings. God punishes evil and rewards good. God will send a Messiah. God will resurrect the dead.
2 **Torah.** The Torah (teaching or direction) is of divine origin. The Torah is eternally valid.
3 **Israel.** Jews must worship God alone. God has communicated through the prophets. Moses is the greatest of the prophets.

The religious precepts are simply to:

- worship one God
- carry out the Ten Commandments
- practise charity and tolerance towards other people.

The British Jewish community identifies with neither a specific country of origin nor a particular ethnic group. However, religion and culture are inextricably mixed. There is a wide variety of beliefs and attitudes, and of languages spoken.

Observant Jews have specific dietary and other religious requirements and may hold cultural beliefs about health, illness, life and death.

There are several different traditions within Judaism, each with its own particular religious observances, namely Hasidic, Ultra-Orthodox, Orthodox, Masorti, Conservative, Progressive, Reform and Liberal Judaism.

Orthodox Judaism consists of two groups, namely the Modern Orthodox, who have integrated into society while still observing the Jewish law, and the Ultra-Orthodox, who live separately and dress in a traditional manner.

Generic practices and requirements are given below with regard to Jewish patients, with special references to a particular tradition being made as necessary.

Keeping the Sabbath

The Sabbath is central to the rhythm of Jewish individual, family and communal life, and is observed as a day of rest and peace. Saturday is believed to correspond to the seventh day, on which God rested from the task of creation. The Sabbath begins half an hour before sunset on Friday and ends at nightfall on Saturday.

During the Sabbath all Jews are forbidden to engage in any activities that can be regarded as work. Each tradition interprets this differently. For example, Orthodox Jews will not drive a car, as this involves making a spark in the engine. By contrast, Progressive Jews do not consider this to be work and therefore do drive on the Sabbath.

The exception to this is in the event of an emergency, when the requirement to sustain life takes precedence over normal Jewish law.

The practical implications for the treatment of Orthodox Jewish patients can be anticipated with some careful preparation in most cases. In circumstances where life is threatened, the requirement to sustain life takes precedence.

- Progressive, Reform and Liberal Jews will not object to taking medication on the Sabbath, and if the condition is serious they will accept non-kosher medication.
- Surgery, tests and other procedures can be scheduled for non-Sabbath or non-holy days.
- Orthodox and Hasidic Jews will expect to maintain a far stricter adherence to the Jewish law.
- All medicines must be kosher (i.e. they must not contain pig products, blood or gelatine).
- The only exception to the use of kosher medicine is if there is immediate danger of death of the patient. Then the duty to save life is the overriding principle.
- If a patient is fasting on a holy day, consider injecting the medication rather than giving a pill or tablet.
- If the patient needs to take medication daily (e.g. a diabetic who uses insulin injections), it is possible for this to be prepared in advance of the Sabbath and stored in the refrigerator until required.
- If a blood test is needed, this will be permitted on the grounds that it is necessary for health, especially in an emergency.

Names

The structure of Jewish names follows the pattern of one or two personal names followed by a surname or family name.

Religious obligations

- Prayer/worship. Three daily prayers are stipulated – in the morning, in the afternoon and in the evening. Communal prayer can take place anywhere, and does not require a Rabbi to officiate.
- In the Orthodox tradition, prayer can only be said when a group of 10 or more Jewish men has been convened.

- During weekday morning prayers, some Jewish men wear Tephillin (phylacteries). These are two leather boxes containing tiny scrolls from the Torah. One is tied to the forehead and the other is bound around the left arm and hand with a leather strap.
- Prayer shawls (Tallitot) may also be worn.
- The Sabbath (Shabbat) begins half an hour before sunset on Friday evening and ends with the first sighting of three stars on Saturday evening, with a blessing for the coming week.
- During Shabbat, Jews are forbidden to engage in any activities that are considered as work. However, this is interpreted in varying ways depending upon the particular Jewish tradition to which the patient belongs and whether the individual actively practises their religion in this respect.
- 'Work 'relates to creative acts, or acts which change one condition into another. For example, a fully observant (Orthodox) Jew is not allowed to switch on or turn off a light, or even to ask someone else to do it for them during Shabbat. However, the person may accept help with this if it is offered. This law also extends to travelling, which may sometimes impact upon discharge planning. Sabbath laws also extend to a prohibition on the carrying of money or gifts, or the purchase of any articles or refreshments.
- Any religious law may be transgressed if life is in danger.
- The Torah (or Pentateuch) is the most important Jewish holy book. The Jewish patient may bring a printed version for hospital use. Synagogues keep copies of the Torah on a parchment scroll which is covered by a mantle when not in use.

Festivals

- Passover/the Festival of Unleavened Bread celebrates the Exodus from Egypt by the Children of Israel. The message is about national and personal freedom. During the festival the diet is strictly 'unleavened' and kosher hospital meals will be in accordance with this practice. No bread must be consumed. Jewish patients may prefer to have food brought from home, especially on the first night when a special meal is eaten. The festival falls at around the same time as the Christian festival of Easter.
- Ten Days of Awe (or repentance for our sins) takes place in the early autumn and commences with two days of the Jewish New Year. The tenth day is the Day of Atonement, which is a solemn 25-hour fast. If a practising Jew is in hospital at this time a doctor must be consulted regarding the fitness of the patient to undertake this fast. Seek advice from a Rabbi of the same tradition if you are unsure.
- Tabernacles (Succoth) begins five days after Yom Kippur and cannot be kept in hospital. Orthodox Jews create temporary structures outdoors in

which they eat their meals, as they remember the protection of the Children of Israel by God.

- A minor festival – Chanukah (Festival of Lights) – takes place in December (sometimes close to Christmas). Candles are lit during this festival, and some patients may wish to display Chanukah lights on the ward. Work is permitted.

During the major festivals the same laws regarding work apply. However, the actual keeping of the festivals will vary depending on the tradition to which a particular Jewish person belongs.

Diet

- Jewish food laws are known as Kashrut (fitness). Food is either permitted (kosher) or forbidden (trief).
- Animals destined for consumption by Jewish people are slaughtered by a qualified Jewish slaughterer. Permitted foods are marked with a seal to show that they are kosher.
- Observant Jews are permitted to eat the following:
  - eggs
  - milk
  - chicken
  - fish (not shellfish)
  - kosher beef
  - kosher lamb
  - yoghurt
  - butter
  - cheese that has no animal content
  - all fruit and vegetables.
- Observant Jews are not permitted to eat the following:
  - pork, shellfish
  - non-kosher meat
  - milk or cheese products or items at or after meat meals. These products may be eaten separately, with a time lapse between their consumption.
- Jewish patients should be informed of the availability of kosher meals. Some may not use this facility and instead choose suitable meals from the standard menu (e.g. fish or vegetarian meals).
- Observant Jews are required to keep the preparation, serving and storage of food separate from that of non-kosher foods and implements. The following practices should be maintained on the wards.
  - Kosher meals should be served with disposable cutlery and should not be removed from their container, or unsealed by staff, or put on hospital plates.
  - There should be no probing to test the temperature of the food.

- Separate sets of kitchen utensils should be used for meat and milk dishes.

Dress

- Some Jewish men may wear a small cap (Kappah).
- Orthodox Jewish men prefer to be bearded or will use only an electric razor (a modern circumvention of a ruling against shaving).
- Some Jewish men may wear a prayer shawl around their waist, under a jacket or outer clothing.
- Some Jewish men may also keep a phylactery (a small box containing portions of scripture) for tying around their head and left arm while praying.
- Married Orthodox Jewish women may keep their hair covered (some women wear a wig to cover their own hair).

Language

Members of Jewish families generally use English as their main language, although Yiddish and Hebrew may also be spoken. Some Jewish people may also speak other European languages.

Birth

- An Orthodox Jewish husband will not touch his wife while she is giving birth, as Jewish teaching indicates that she is unclean at this time, due to the loss of blood.
- Within the Reformed, Progressive and Liberal traditions this prohibition in relation to touching would not be supported.
- Baby boys are circumcised on the eighth day after birth. The operation is postponed in the event of infantile jaundice, premature birth or any other contraindications.
- The circumcision ceremony is usually performed at home, although it can take place in hospital.
- The birth of a daughter simply requires the giving of a name.
- Among Orthodox Jews, baby girls are given their name on the Sabbath after the birth, whereas boys are named after the circumcision ceremony.
- Among Reform and Progressive Jews, both boys and girls have baby-blessing ceremonies, which are normally held during the Sabbath morning services in the Synagogue.

Orthodox Jewish attitudes to miscarriage and stillbirth

- Prior to 30 days' gestation a fetus is not accorded any status as a person. If there is a miscarriage, there is no religious requirement for any prayers or a funeral. Only after a fetus has reached 30 days' gestation is it considered to have had a 'breath of life', and it should then be treated as having been a living person.
- When a fetus has reached 40 days' gestation or more but has been miscarried, the tissue must be collected and buried. The parents must be consulted about their wishes for disposal. Although the fetus must be buried, cremation of the non-fetal tissue is permitted.
- While some Orthodox Jews do not give full recognition to a stillborn baby, there will be exceptions to this rule. Parents must be offered the opportunity to hold the baby. Some Orthodox men whose families are descended from the priesthood, and who are not allowed to be near dead bodies, may have to leave the room.
- The parents may wish the baby's body to be laid out in the traditional Jewish manner prior to burial. Unless the parents specify otherwise, the Jewish Burial Society must be contacted so that they may attend to the necessary arrangements.
- The mourning period (Shivah) may not be observed.

Reform Jewish attitudes to miscarriage and stillbirth

- Reform Judaism recognises that the loss of a child, at any age of gestation, can cause profound distress to the parents and to other members of the family. This tradition recognises a need to give some formal expression to their grief.
- Although no funeral will take place, it is possible for a Rabbi to conduct a simple service in the home, if the parents request this.
- Reform Judaism recognises the trauma that stillbirth causes for the parents and extended family.
- It is possible for parents to acknowledge the loss by holding a funeral. The baby is placed in its own grave following a simple funeral service that is mainly attended by the immediate family.
- A shortened period of mourning (Shivah) may also take place, followed by the erection of a headstone with the child's name inscribed on it.

Personal hygiene

Jews are expected to wash their hands and to say a prayer before eating. There are no other specific religious requirements with regard to personal hygiene.

Gender, privacy and dignity

- Jewish patients prefer to be accommodated in single-sex wards or bays.
- Orthodox Jewish women will prefer female medical staff to examine them.
- Ultra-Orthodox Jews consider it immodest to touch women other than their wives.
- Orthodox Jewish patients may object to female Rabbis.

Attitude to illness

- In a medical emergency the Sabbath laws are set aside, as the saving of life takes precedence over the keeping of the laws.
- Jewish people treat the medical profession with respect while at the same time being prepared to ask pertinent questions related to their condition.

Blood transfusions

There are no objections to blood transfusions.

Religious implications of menstruation

- Within the Orthodox Jewish tradition, women are considered to be unclean during menstruation. Physical contact of any kind between husband and wife is prohibited at this time.
- Within the Reform, Liberal and Progressive Jewish traditions this prohibition does not apply, although individual adherence will vary.
- Mikveh is ritual cleansing in water, which traditionally takes place after menstruation and marks the regaining of a woman's bodily rhythm after her period. A Mikveh is a small pool that is usually located adjacent to the Synagogue.
- Within Orthodox Judaism it is expected that a woman will attend the Mikveh each month.
- Within the more liberal traditions this ritual is not obligatory, although some women may choose to adhere to it. This may be associated more with a discovery of the Jewish feminist movement and the search for female customs and rituals than with having a relationship with the traditional Jewish concept of Mikveh.

Contraception

- Almost all Jews use some method of family planning.
- Orthodox Jews favour large families and may be reluctant to use contraception. Couples may wish to consult with a Rabbi about this.
- Abortion is permitted only in emergencies, when the pregnancy presents a physical or mental risk to the woman.

- Abortion is permitted in the case of a pregnancy arising from rape or incest.
- It is preferable for the termination to take place within the first 40 days of the pregnancy.

Orthodox Jewish attitudes to fertility treatment

There is a strong religious emphasis upon a woman's fertility, with many Orthodox Jewish families being large. Where these hopes and expectations are not met, the distress experienced by the husband and wife is immense. Jewish women who ovulate early in the cycle may be at greater risk of not conceiving if they keep the law regarding the avoidance of sexual intercourse within the first 7 days following a menstrual period. In these circumstances a couple may choose to use artificial insemination during this time, rather than break the law. However, other methods for the collection of sperm and for insemination during this time may be considered. Artificial insemination using another man's sperm would be unacceptable on religious grounds. In the same way the use of donated eggs would also be unacceptable. However, IVF using the couple's own eggs and sperm may be acceptable.

Visiting

- Visiting of the sick is regarded as an important religious duty, and Jewish patients may receive many visitors.
- For Orthodox Jews on the Sabbath and during major festivals visiting may be more limited, unless the visitors are able to walk to the hospital.
- The Sabbath rules are lifted when a patient is dying.
- Members of the Jewish community are also happy to visit any Jewish patients who do not have family or friends in the area.
- The Jewish Visitation Committee selects and trains Jewish people for visiting the sick in hospital, and can be contacted for details of approved visitors in the locality.

Orthodox Jewish requirements during dying and death

- A dying person should not be left alone, but must have someone sitting with them at all times.
- Jewish law prohibits any active intervention that would hasten the death of a terminally ill person. Where any ethical/religious question arises in this respect, a Rabbi should be consulted.
- In Orthodox Jewish law the moving or touching of a dying person is not permitted. The giving of pain relief is permitted.
- A dying patient may wish to recite the 'Shema' or special psalms as well as a deathbed confession known as the 'Vidui'. They may appreciate being able to hold the page on which it is written.

- Most patients will wish to see their own Rabbi or the Jewish Chaplain.
- Orthodox and Hasidic Jews may not accept brain death as a definition of death. The traditional understanding is that the body has to be without breath or heartbeat for a short period of time, which would then make resuscitation impossible. Some Jews may wish to use a traditional method in which a feather is placed over the nose and mouth of the deceased person as a means of detecting any breath.
- Following the death the relatives may request a Rabbi, or their local synagogue, to be contacted so that the last rites may be performed.
- If these individuals cannot be contacted, healthcare staff are permitted to perform any essential procedures as follows.
  - Close the eyes and mouth.
  - Catheters, drains and tubes should be left *in situ*, as fluid contained within them is considered to be part of the body and must be kept with it ready for burial. They may be covered with gauze or bandages.
  - Open wounds must be covered.
  - Lay out the body flat, with the hands open, the arms parallel and close to the body, and the legs stretched out straight.
  - Try to make sure that someone stays with the body (if there are no relatives) until a member of the Jewish Burial Society arrives.
  - Do not wash the body, as the Jewish Burial Society will do this. It will be a ritual washing (Taharah).
  - If death occurs on the Sabbath, the body must be removed to the mortuary until the end of the Sabbath. This consideration will also apply on Jewish holy days. Some Orthodox Jews insist on keeping watch in close proximity to the body at all times, and may request that they be allowed to sit in or near the mortuary area.
  - Traditionally the body is covered with a plain white sheet and laid on the floor, with the feet pointing towards the door.
  - A lit candle may be placed near the head.
- If the relatives are present, the son (or the nearest relative) will prepare the body as described above.
- Some families may ask to keep a vigil and remain with or near the body, to pray. This may include staying near the body while it is in the mortuary. This tradition has practical origins – vachers (watchers) were used to keep the body safe from body snatchers and rodents.
- There is a mourning period of seven days following the death.
- Jewish law requires burial to take place as soon as possible after death. Any unnecessary delay must be avoided.

Reform Jewish requirements during dying and death

- Reform Jews do not prohibit the touching of a corpse by non-Jews. The ban on the touching of dead bodies by non-Jews relates to historic pagan practices of corpse mutilation. Reform Jews support the after-death care for a Jewish patient being provided by non-Jewish health-care staff.

- The ritual washing of the body (Taharah) will be undertaken either by trained members of the Synagogue or by the Jewish Burial Society.
- Cremation is permitted within the non-Orthodox Jewish communities, and is being increasingly used for strong theological as well as environmental reasons.

Post-mortem

- Orthodox Jewish law does not allow a post-mortem, except in an emergency or in cases where civil law requires it. The procedure is considered to be a desecration of the body, and emphasis is given to maintaining the physical integrity of the body whatever the cost.
- If a post-mortem is essential, it is good practice for the Rabbi to be able to liaise with the Coroner.
- Reform, Liberal and Progressive Jews permit post-mortems on the grounds that medical knowledge gained from them can be of benefit in the treatment of other people.

Practical considerations with regard to post-mortem for Orthodox Jews
- Place the body on a clean white cloth so that all bodily fluids escape into the cloth.
- Unnecessary damage to the body must be avoided.
- The body must not be placed face down and, if possible, it must be kept covered.
- Samples taken from the body must be as minimal as possible.
- Wherever possible, incisions should be avoided.
- After the procedure all organs must be returned to the body, in their natural location if possible.
- The cloth must also be packed into the body.

Organ and tissue donation

- Organ donation may be permitted when the organ is needed for a specific and immediate transplant.
- Jewish law does not support the donation of organs for general medical research or to an organ bank.
- In principle, Judaism supports and encourages organ donation in order to save lives. This principle can sometimes override the strong objections to any unnecessary interference with the body after death, and the requirement for immediate burial of the complete body.

Orthodox considerations with regard to organ and tissue donation
- Orthodox authorities permit organ donations only when there is a recipient who needs the organ(s) in order to survive.

- In general, Orthodox Jews support the receipt of blood, blood products, bone marrow, corneas and kidneys. In Jewish law a doctor is obliged to screen donors before using donated blood, tissue or organs.
- For some Jews it is crucial for a person to be buried with the body intact. In such circumstances organ donation would be insupportable except in the case of blood, blood products and bone marrow, all of which are replaced naturally.

Reform considerations with regard to organ and tissue donation

- The Reform tradition supports the taking of organs in cases where there is not a specific recipient, but where there would be a use for the organs in the future.
- Similarly, the use of organs that can improve the quality of life, but not save it (e.g. eyes for corneal transplants), is supported by the Reform tradition.
- The donation of organs or tissue from a living person (e.g. a lung or a kidney, or bone marrow) is also permitted only in circumstances where it would not endanger the life of the donor.
- A Jew may receive the organs/tissues of another Jew, or of a non-Jew, which will enhance or save his or her life. This would also apply to the use of non-kosher animal organs (e.g. a pig's heart) for human transplant. The overriding principle is that the saving of life is more important than the keeping of a particular law.

Pagan

Background and beliefs

Paganism is a religion in its own right, and can be traced from prehistoric times through most ancient and modern cultures. Paganism believes in a divine creative force. It is principally rooted in the old religions of Europe, although some adherents also find great worth in the indigenous beliefs of other countries. Pagans believe in the sacredness of all things.

Pagans honour the divine in all its aspects, whether male or female. The essential personification of the divine creative force focuses upon the male and female aspects – the Mother Goddess and the Father God. The Goddess represents nourishing, synthesising and intuitive aspects, and the Father God represents the fertilising, energising, analysing and intellectual capacities. Such characteristics manifest themselves throughout the created order.

Pagans do not worship the devil. Evil is regarded as an imbalance to be corrected, and not as an independent force or entity.

Pagans make use of many different Goddess and God forms as 'tuning signals' to different aspects of the essential Goddess and God. These forms vary according to cultural, geographical and personal circumstances, and are usually envisaged in perfected human form.

Pagans believe in a multi-level reality perceived as spiritual, mental (or rational), ethical, astral and physical. Each has its own laws, which are not in conflict with one another.

Pagan philosophy and worship tend to be nature based. Mother Earth is understood as being a home, for whose well-being and protection we bear a responsibility. Pagan worship rites help believers to harmonise with natural cycles, so they are usually held at the turning points of the seasons – at the phases of the sun and moon – and at times of transition in our lives.

There is a great diversity within Paganism, which reflects the range of spiritual experience. Some Pagans follow multiple Gods and Goddesses, some focus on a single Life Force of no or specific gender, while others devote themselves to a 'cosmic couple' – Lord and Lady, God and Goddess.

Most Pagans believe in reincarnation. This is viewed as being a moral force, as it emphasises that all offences against other individuals, the community or the earth, and all failure to learn lessons must be put right by each individual, and that this responsibility cannot be evaded by physical death.

Paganism's positive ethical attitude is summed up as follows: 'Do what you will, and harm no one.'

The Pagan Federation is an umbrella organisation with a membership drawn from all strands within Paganism.

Names

Some Pagans have a name that they take on becoming a Pagan. However, this name is not always used in normal circumstances, so an individual may not refer to it during any hospital admission.

Religious obligations

There are no specific obligations. Many Pagans follow an eight-fold yearly festival pattern:

1 Early February – Imbolc: The celebration of the re-awakening of the earth. These celebrations include the Goddes Bride, or Brigid, the Goddess of Light and of the hearth.
2 Spring Equinox: This celebration takes place around 21 March and remembers the Goddess Oestara, a fertility goddess who crossed the land leaving tokens of fertility (eggs, and her totem animal, the hare). The Church absorbed this into its own culture and religion, keeping Easter, with traditional Easter eggs, and the Easter bunny. Some Pagans may re-enact a battle between the Oak King who rules the summer, and the Holly King who rules the winter.
3 Beltaine (May Day): This is a celebration of fertility when the young God and Goddess come together. Bonfires and May crowns characterise this festival, although some Pagans do not agree with maypoles since they regard this as a Victorian invention. Originally farmers used to drive their cattle between two bonfires to assure fertility. Sometimes couples will jump a bonfire for the same reason.
4 Summer Solstice (around 21 June): This is the time of year when the Sun is at its strongest and the God is at the height of his rule. Some celebrate the battle of Oak and Holly, but many reserve this battle for the two equinoxes.
5 Lughnassadh: This is the feast of the God Lugh – a God of light – and takes place in early August. The festival celebrates the first fruits of the harvest. Tradition tells of the Corn Lord taking up the fears of his people into himself and becoming the willing sacrifice who gives up his life for the good of his land.
6 Autumn Equinox (around 21 September): This celebrates the end of harvest and the return battle between Oak and Holly.
7 Samhain: This is a feast of remembrance, when the veil between the worlds becomes thin and people may receive messages from their departed loved ones. This festival places emphasis upon our human mortality, as well as kindling a hope for a time of rest and recreation before rebirth.
8 Winter Solstice (around 21 December): This feast is known as Yule and celebrates the fact that the longest night is over and that the daylight will once more begin to lengthen. Traditionally it is the festival of the

rebirth of the God who was conceived at Beltaine, whose father died at Lughnassadh. There is a continuous cycle of death and rebirth throughout the Pagan year which is reflected in the smaller cycles of loss/death and renewal of life in our individual lives.

Pagans usually acknowledge the phases of the moon, of which the phase of the full moon is the most important. This is followed by the dark moon (when the moon is not seen in the sky). The first and last quarters of the moon's phases are less acknowledged.

Diet

Some Pagans are vegetarians or vegans. Others fast for personal reasons. There are no religious requirements that govern diet in general.

Dress

- No specific dress is required for a Pagan.
- Most Pagans wear symbolic jewellery that relates to their particular spiritual path. Care should be taken whenever the jewellery needs to be removed for medical reasons, and it should be returned to the person as soon as possible.

Language

Paganism is culturally and ethnically diverse.

Birth

- Birth is viewed as sacred and empowering. It is possible that Pagan women may choose not to have much pain relief, seeking to manage the pain in other ways.
- Pagan women will wish to make their own informed decisions about pre- and postnatal care.
- There are no religious requirements, but individual Pagans may have particular wishes to be considered (e.g. naming ceremonies).

Gender, privacy and dignity

There are no specific needs. In general, Pagans are relaxed about medical examinations.

Attitude to illness

- Most Pagans practise complementary therapies alongside conventional medical treatments.
- Some Pagan patients may welcome a healing ritual performed for them by Pagans who are able to do this.
- Some Pagans will regard illness as a trial set by their Gods on their road to enlightenment.

- Pagans may choose to make a Living Will and will wish to be fully informed of their condition and to make shared decisions about their treatment with healthcare professionals. Some Pagans may request that there is no intervention.

Blood transfusions

There are no religious objections to blood transfusions.

Contraception

- There are no religious objections to contraception, which is a private matter for individual couples to decide. However, pregnancies are usually planned.
- Paganism emphasises women's control over their own bodies. Women take the lead in making these decisions and are supported in the choices that they make.

Fertility treatment

There is no general prohibition regarding fertility treatment and each couple will require specific attention.

Visiting

Pagans will naturally wish for members of their Pagan community to visit them in hospital.

Dying and death

- Pagans accept dying as part of the cycle of life, and most believe in reincarnation.
- Pagan patients will wish to know when they are dying, so that they may prepare for death.
- Rituals may take the form of 'last rites' performed by one or more Pagan members to help the spirit of the dying person to go into transition peacefully.
- If the patient or their family do not have someone specific they can ask to do this, the Pagan Federation will be able to assist.
- After death there is no requirement for the body to be dressed in particular clothes, although relatives and friends may have specific requirements.
- Some families will wish to take the body home to prepare it for burial or cremation themselves, while others will employ a funeral director.

Post-mortem

There are no religious objections to post-mortem, although individuals may express particular preferences.

Organ and tissue donation

There are no religious objections to this, although individuals may express particular preferences.

Sikh

Background and beliefs

Sikhism originated in the Punjab about 500 years ago, and was founded by Guru Nanak, who envisaged a society in which every member would work for the common good. The word 'Sikh' means discipline. Guru Nanak drew on aspects of Hinduism and Islam to create a reformist movement. He and nine other Gurus who followed him sought to set an example of living spiritually while at the same time taking an active part in the world.

Sikhs believe in one God (the eternal source of light and creator of all being) and in many cycles of rebirth. They respect the equality of all people, regardless of caste, colour, creed or sex.

Sikhism supports and encourages free belief and the pursuit of knowledge. Followers are encouraged to make the most of opportunities in life, in order to achieve union with God through truthful conduct, humility, family life, meditation and prayer. Emphasis and encouragement are given to the service of the community. This service may include the giving of money, clothing, food and shelter to those in need. Failure in this service is believed to affect the cycle of rebirth.

The spiritual message taught by Guru Nanak has three elements:

1 meditation, which now includes chanting hymns composed by the Gurus
2 honest toil – earning a living by honest means
3 sharing – giving to the poor and needy, and contributing one-tenth of one's income to good causes.

There are around 300 000 Sikhs living in the UK. One can either be born into a Sikh family or choose to become a Sikh.

Names

- Many Sikh names are unisex, gender being differentiated by the shared middle name to illustrate the unity of all and the eradication of caste.
- All Sikh men have the second name Singh, meaning 'lion.' All Sikh women have the middle name Kaur, meaning 'princess.' These middle names must not be confused with surnames.
- Sikhs usually prefer to be called by their first name, or by their first name and middle name (Singh or Kaur). To avoid confusion in medical records, it is best to use the family name or surname.
- Young Asians follow the western practice of using only their first and last names.

Religious obligations

- As an act of faith, baptised Sikhs wear the five K's.
  1 Kesh – uncut hair. Men wear their long hair under a turban. Women wear their hair either loose or tied back. For both men and women uncut hair symbolises sanctity and a love of nature.
  2 Kangha – a wooden comb symbolising cleanliness. It is worn above the man's top-knot, and above the woman's bun or plait.
  3 Kara – a steel bangle worn on the right wrist. It symbolises strength and restraint and is a visual link with the Gurus.
  4 Kirpan – a short sword or dagger symbolising the readiness of the Sikh to fight against injustice and to protect the oppressed. It is often worn on a cotton body belt underneath the clothes.
  5 Kaccha – a particular design of unisex undershorts with a drawstring waist. It symbolises sexual morality.
- It is important to respect the Sikh patient's need to wear the five K's, unless it is necessary for them to be removed for medical purposes.
- Nowadays most Sikhs wear only the Kesh and the Kara. Many third-generation Sikhs choose to have short hair.
- Healthcare staff should consider offering an alternative head covering to male Sikh patients pre-operatively. Equally, it may not always be necessary for the male patient to be shaved pre-operatively, thereby avoiding the shaving of the beard or cutting of long hair.
- Daily prayers are said in the early morning, at sunset and before going to sleep. These prayers may be said privately, or with other Sikhs.
- Sikh patients will have a smaller version of the holy book (the Guru Granth Sahib), called the Gutka, which contains the morning and evening prayers. It is wrapped in a clean cloth and should be kept in a clean place.
- A patient who is too ill to recite the hymns or prayers should be allowed to listen to an audiotape, or to have a relative read them aloud.

Diet

- Sikhs are forbidden to eat Halal, kosher or beef. Some Sikh women may prefer to eat no meat at all.
- Sikhs prefer to eat chicken, lamb, pork and fish.
- Some Sikhs are vegetarians.
- Vegetarian Sikhs do not eat fish or eggs.
- It is important not to use the same utensils to cook for Sikhs as have been used to cook or store Halal, kosher or beef.
- There are no specific times for fasting, although some Sikhs may wish to fast when there is a full moon.
- Most Sikhs do not smoke or drink alcohol.

Dress

- Many male Sikh patients will wear a smaller version of the turban to cover their hair while in hospital.
- Removing the turban without permission, except in an emergency, is considered an insult.
- There is no restriction on what women may wear. However, female Sikhs will tend to wear Punjabi female dress consisting of loose trousers and a tunic, with a headscarf (Shalwar-Kamees and a dupatta).

Language

- Members of Sikh families in the UK may speak several languages other than English.
- In general, Punjabi is most commonly spoken by Sikhs, and sometimes Swahili. Punjabi speakers may also understand Urdu and Hindi to some extent.

Birth

- There are no religious practices associated with birth.
- Relatives will be keen to visit the mother and baby as soon as possible after the birth, bringing with them gifts of clothes for the new arrival.
- Relatives will be concerned to allow the mother complete rest for 40 days after giving birth. This attitude is based on the belief that a woman is at her weakest at this time.

Personal hygiene

- Sikhism emphasises cleanliness.
- Sikhs prefer to wash in free-flowing water. Thus showers are preferred to baths.
- Running water is needed for washing after using the toilet or bedpan.
- Sikhs prefer to brush their teeth and wash their face and hands before eating and drinking.

Gender, privacy and dignity

- Sikhism teaches that all people are equal.
- Men and women enjoy equal status within this religion.
- Culturally, women may adopt a subservient role in public.
- Within the family, the mother-in-law or the oldest woman has significant power. This may affect the choices open to younger women in the family.

- Healthcare staff should seek to reinforce the autonomy of Sikh women in any decision making.
- Sikh women prefer to be examined by female doctors. In emergencies they do not mind being examined by male doctors so long as there is a female staff member present.
- Accommodation in single-sex wards is essential.
- Hospital gowns should be of sufficient length to avoid embarrassment.

Attitude to illness

Generally speaking, members of the Sikh community are willing to accept the authority of the professional healthcare staff. However, they may be slow to seek medical advice in the first instance.

Blood transfusions

There are no objections to blood transfusions.

Contraception

- Sikhism encourages large families.
- Contraceptives are not prohibited, and most methods are acceptable.
- Termination of a pregnancy is not supported, except in cases where the mother's health is in danger.

Miscarriage, stillbirth and neonatal death

- If a late miscarriage occurs, the baby should be given to the parents for the fulfilment of the funeral rites.
- Stillborn babies and those who die in the neonatal period may be buried.

Fertility treatment

Fertility treatment is generally acceptable to Sikhs. However, there may be reluctance to use donor eggs or sperm.

Visiting

- It is a Sikh custom for family, friends and other members of the community to visit sick relatives. This is seen to be an act of faith and part of family life. It may be helpful to allow some easing of any regulations limiting the number of people who can visit the bedside at any one time.

- Elderly patients will have particular need of visitors for moral support and reassurance.

Dying and death

- A dying Sikh may derive comfort from reciting verses, or having them recited to him or her, from the holy book (the Guru Granth Sahib).
- Patients or relatives may request the service of a Sikh priest (granthi) during the last stages of the patient's life.
- Holy water from the Gurdwara may be given to the patient to sip, or it may be sprinkled on or around the patient.
- If no relatives are present at the time of death, they should be contacted as soon as possible.
- The relatives may wish to prepare the body, but it should not be assumed that this is the case.
- Non-Sikhs are allowed to touch the body, and healthcare staff may perform the last offices.
- The five K's must be left on the body.
- The body of the deceased should be covered with a plain white sheet.
- The body must not be sent to the hospital mortuary before any relatives arrive.
- The body may be handled by hospital staff, with due regard for the patient's requirement to be touched/attended to by healthcare staff of the same gender.
- The mouth and the eyes must be closed.
- Make sure that the patient's face is clean and straightened as necessary.
- Straighten the limbs, placing the arms by the side of the body.
- Sikh faith requires that the funeral should take place as quickly as possible after death, if there are no legal requirements for a post-mortem.
- Sikh faith and custom require cremation of the body.

Post-mortem

There are no religious objections to post-mortems, although Sikhs prefer the body to remain intact.

Organ and tissue donation

- Sikhs believe that life after death is a continuous cycle of rebirth, but that the physical body is not needed for this, as a person's soul is their real essence.
- Sikh philosophy and teachings place great emphasis on the importance of giving and of putting others before oneself. It also stresses the importance of performing noble deeds. Within this context there is no objection to organ and tissue donation.

Zoroastrian

Background and beliefs

Zarathushtra was a prophet who founded Zoroastrianism, and lived in Eastern Iran around 6000 BC. Zarathushtra (the Greek name is Zoroaster) proclaimed the worship of Ahura Mazda (the Wise Lord or the Lord of Wisdom), who is believed to have created a good world consisting of seven elements of creation, namely the sky, waters, earth, plants, cattle, humans and fire.

In the tenth century a group of Zoroastrians settled in India and became known as Parsis, where the majority lived in Bombay and Gujarat state.

Zarathushtra saw the world as a theatre of conflict between two opposed moral spirits – the Spirit of Goodness and the Spirit of Evil. The highest form of existence is Asha Vahishta (highest truth and righteousness). Each person possesses Vohu-Mana (the quality of the good mind). This enables people to lay hold of Asha and to see how any part of the world may deviate from this. There is a general movement from right thoughts to right actions known as the Spirit of Piety or Devotion. The three-way pattern of Zoroastrian devotion is as follows:

1 good thoughts – humata
2 good words – hukhta
3 good deeds – hvarshta.

Zoroastrians are encouraged to live life to the full while engaging in ethical, honest and charitable activities.

The consequences of right actions lead to the establishment of the ideal society, of the kingdom of heaven. The person who lives in this way achieves a state of well-being. On dying the person enters into a state of immortal bliss.

Names

- Each Zoroastrian has three names – a given name, the father's forename and a family name or surname that may also indicate a profession.
- When a woman marries or remarries, the middle name is changed to that of her husband.

Religious obligations

- Before prayers, Zoroastrians will wash their hands, face and other uncovered parts of their body.

- The day is divided into five periods – sunrise to noon, noon to 3.00pm, 3.00pm to sunset, sunset to midnight, and midnight to sunrise.
- The Kushti (the sacred cord) will be untied and held before a source of light.
- Two prayers are said, preferably in a prayer room, or in privacy behind closed bed curtains.

Diet

There are no restrictions concerning diet or alcohol. However, due to personal choice some Zoroastrians will not eat pork or beef, and some are vegetarian.

Dress

Zoroastrians are required to wear two items of clothing at all times.

1 Sudreh – a white sacred shirt made of muslin or cotton that symbolises purity and good deeds.
2 Kushti – a sacred cord woven from 72 threads of fine lambswool. This symbolises the 72 chapters of the Yasna (Act of Worship), and is worn over the Sudreh.

Language

- Zoroastrians belong to what is now a dispersed community, with members settling in different parts of the world. Thus they may speak any one of a number of languages as well as English.
- An interpreter may occasionally be required.

Birth

- There are no specific religious requirements with regard to the birth of a baby.
- Parsi children are admitted into the faith at a ceremony called 'Navjote', between the ages of 7 and 15 years. The Sudreh and the Kushti are put on for the first time during this ceremony.

Personal hygiene

- Running water for washing is essential, as Zoroastrians have very high standards of hygiene.
- A bowl of fresh water at the bedside is appreciated.

Gender, privacy and dignity

The same considerations apply here as for all other patients, particularly Asian patients.

Attitude to illness

Parsees (Indian Zoroastrians) have adapted to western ways and thus accept western medication and treatments.

Blood transfusions

Zoroastrians may not accept blood transfusions. Therefore it is advisable to consult the patient and/or their relatives before proceeding.

Contraception

There are no specific religious objections to contraception.

Fertility treatment

There is no general objection to fertility treatment on religious grounds. However, careful consideration should be given to couples who practice this religion.

Visiting

- Zoroastrian patients will welcome visits by relatives and other members of the community.
- Prayers may be said and portions of the holy book may be read aloud.

Dying and death

According to the Zoroastrian creed, at death the soul is earthbound for three days. Because of this it is necessary to begin prayers for the dead person as soon as possible.

- If there are no relatives present, another Zoroastrian must be contacted.
- The body must be washed before being dressed in white clothing.
- A special Sudreh and Kushta must be worn under the shroud, next to the skin.
- The head may be covered by a cap or a scarf.
- The family may wish to prepare the body for the funeral, but this task is usually performed by the funeral director.

- Cremation and burial are both acceptable.
- The reasons for any potential delays to the funeral must be clearly explained.

Post-mortem

Religious law prohibits post-mortems except for legal reasons.

Organ and tissue donation

- Orthodox Zoroastrians consider the pollution of the body to be contrary to the will of God. Within this context there are religious objections to organ and tissue donation.
- Less Orthodox Zoroastrians may take a different approach to this issue and should be consulted.

Further reading

Akhtar S (2002) Nursing with dignity. Part 8. Islam. *Nurs Times.* **98(16):** 40–2.

Baxter C (2002) Nursing with dignity. Part 5. Rastafarianism. *Nurs Times.* **98(13):** 42–3.

Chaplaincy and Pastoral Care Department, Epsom and St Helier NHS Trust. *World Faiths in Hospital* (3e). Chaplaincy and Pastoral Care Department, Epsom and St Helier NHS Trust, Surrey.

Christmas M (2002) Nursing with dignity. Part 3. Christianity I. *Nurs Times.* **98(11):** 37–9.

Cobb M and Robshaw V (eds) (1998) *The Spiritual Challenge of Healthcare.* Elsevier, London.

Collins A (2002) Nursing with dignity. Part 1. Judaism. *Nurs Times.* **98(9):** 33–5.

Department of Spiritual and Religious Care, Bradford Teaching Hospitals NHS Trust (2002) *Faith Requirements Resource Pack. A guide for hospital staff to improve patient care.* Department of Spiritual and Religious Care, Bradford Teaching Hospitals NHS Trust, Bradford.

Faith Regen UK in conjunction with Faith in London (FiL) (2002) *Faith Communities Toolkit. A resource proposed for use within Jobcentreplus.* Faith Regen UK in conjunction with Faith in London (FiL), London.

Gill BK (2002) Nursing with dignity. Part 6. Sikhism. *Nurs Times.* **98(14):** 39–41.

Jogee M and Lal S (1999) *Religions and Cultures. A guide to beliefs and customs for health staff and social care services.* Edinburgh and Lothians Racial Equality Council, Edinburgh.

Jootun D (2002) Nursing with dignity. Part 7. Hinduism. *Nurs Times.* **98(15):** 38–40.

Karmi G (ed.) (1992) *The Ethnic Health Factfile: a guide for health professionals who care for people from ethnic backgrounds.* Health and Ethnicity Programme, Edinburgh.

Lawson R (2003) *Religious and Cultural Needs.* Barnet and Chase Farm NHS Trust, Herts.

Northcott N (2002) Nursing with dignity. Part 2. Buddhism. *Nurs Times.* **98(10):** 36–8.

Orchard O (ed.) (2001) *Spirituality in Healthcare Contexts.* Jessica Kingsley Publishers, London.

Papadopoulos I (2002) Nursing with dignity. Part 4. Christianity II. *Nurs Times.* **98(12):** 36–7.

Romain J (1991) *Faith and Practice. a guide to Reform Judaism today.* Reform Synagogues of Great Britain, London.

Schott J and Henley A (1996) *Culture, Religion and Childbearing in a Multiracial Society. A handbook for health professionals.* Butterworth–Heinemann, Oxford.

Schott J and Henley A (1999) *Culture, Religion and Patient Care in a Multi-Ethnic Society. A handbook for professionals.* Age Concern Books, London.

Sheikh A and Rashid Gatrad A (eds) (2000) *Caring for Muslim Patients*. Radcliffe Medical Press, Oxford.

Simpson J (2002) Nursing with dignity. Part 9. Jehovah's Witnesses. *Nurs Times*. **98(17):** 36–7.

Weller P (ed.) (2001) *Religions in the UK Directory 2001–03*. University of Derby, Derby.

Resources

This chapter provides further information about the UK's cultural and spiritual diversity, faith communities and support organisations.

General

Guide to the Religions of the World; www.bbc.co.uk/worldservice/people/features/world_religions/

Commission for Racial Equality; www.cre.gov.uk

Religions in the UK, a multi-faith directory published by the University of Derby in association with the Interfaith Network for the UK. Can be purchased directly from the University of Derby, Multi-Faith Centre, Kedleston Road, Derby DE22 2GB.

Inter Faith Network for the UK, 5–7 Tavistock Place, London WC1H 9SN; www.interfaith.org.uk

Equality and Diversity; www.dit.gov.uk/er/equality

The Faithworks Campaign; www.faithworkscampaign.org

Ethnicity Online (cultural awareness in healthcare); www.ethnicityonline.net

Spiritual care

Multi-faith Group for Healthcare Chaplaincy; www.mfghc.com

National Chaplaincy Strategy ('Caring for the Spirit'); www.sysha.nhs.uk

Spirituality at work

Future Business Network; www.futurebusiness.org.uk

The Grubb Institute; www.grubb.org.uk

Spirituality at Work; www.spiritualityatwork.com

Your Soul at Work; www.job-search-career.com

Research

Picker Institute Europe (provides newsletter on improvements to services within healthcare by using patient feedback); www.pickereurope.org

Positively Diverse (provides practical advice and guidance on caring for patients from various cultural backgrounds); www.doh.gov.uk/pdfs.posdivfast.pdf

Shrine (provides essential support and networking to all NHS employers, and has produced a handbook to accompany the Positively Diverse process); www.shrine.nhs.uk

Faith organisations in the UK

Baha'i

Baha'i; www.bahai.org
National Spiritual Assembly of the Baha'is of the United Kingdom, 27 Rutland
    Gate, London SW17 1PD. Tel: 0207 584 2566.

Buddhist

Buddhist Society; www.buddsoc.org.uk
Network of Buddhist Organisations UK, The Old Courthouse, 42 Renfrew Road,
    Kennington, London SE11 4NA. Tel: 0208 682 3442.
Friends of the Western Buddhist Order; www.fwbo.org

Christian

Church of England; www.c-of-e.org.uk
Council of Christians and Jews; www.jcrelations.com/ccjuk
Churches Together in Britain and Ireland; www.ctbi.org.uk
Churches Together in England, 27 Tavistock Square, London WC1H 9HH. Tel:
    0207 529 8141; www.churches-together.org.uk
Hospital Chaplaincies Council, Church House, Great Smith Street, London SW1P
    3NZ. Tel: 0207 898 1893.
Roman Catholic Church in England and Wales, 39 Eccleston Square, London
    SW1V 1BX; www.catholic.ew.org.uk
Greek Orthodox Church, Thyateira House, 5 Craven House, London W2 3EN. Tel:
    0207 723 4787.

Hindu

Hindu Council (UK), 74 Llanover Road, North Wembley HA9 7LT. Tel: 07779
    583066; www.hinduforum.org

Islam

Muslim Council of Britain, PO Box 52, Wembley HA9 0XW. Tel: 0208 903 9024;
    www.mcb.org.uk
Sheikh A and Rashid Gatrad A (eds) (2000) *Caring for Muslim Patients*. Radcliffe
    Medical Press, Oxford.

Jain

Institute of Jainology, Unit 18, Silicon Business Centre, 26–28 Wandsworth Road,
    Greenford UB6 7JZ. Tel: 0208 997 2300.

Jehovah's Witness

Jehovah's Witnesses, Hospital Information Services, IBSA House, The Ridgeway, London NW7 1RN. Tel: 0208 906 2211; email: his@wtbts.org.uk
Free Minds; www.freeminds.org
Watchtower News; www.watchtowernews.org
Associated Jehovah's Witnesses for Reform on Blood; www.ajwrb.org

Jewish

Jewish Visitation Committee, United Synagogue, 8/10 Forty Avenue, Wembley HA9 8JW. Tel: 0208 385 1855.
Jewish Burial Society; www.jbs.org.uk
United Society Burial Society. Tel: 0208 343 3456.
Jewish Community Information. Tel: 0207 543 5421.
The Board of Deputies of British Jews. Tel: 0208 543 5400.
Jewish Bereavement Counselling Service. Tel: 0208 349 0839.
Drugsline Chabad (support line for drug users, former users and their relatives). Tel: 0208 518 6470.
Miyad (Jewish crisis helpline). Tel: 08457 581 999.
Chai Lifeline Cancer Care (Jewish Cancer support service). Tel: 0208 202 2211.
Jewish Association for the Mentally Ill. Tel: 0208 458 2223.
London School of Jewish Studies, Schaller House, Albert Road, Hendon, London NW4 1TE. Tel: 0208 203 6427.
Reform Synagogues of Great Britain, The Sternberg Centre for Judaism, 80 East End Road, Finchley, London N3 2SY. Tel: 0208 349 5700; www.reform judaism.org.uk

Pagan

The Pagan Federation, BM Box 7097, London WC1N 3XX; www.paganfed.demon.co.uk
The LifeRites Group, Gwndwn Mawr, Trelech, Carmarthenshire SA33 6SA. Tel: 01994 484527; www.LifeRites.org
The LifeRites group is a UK organisation that is able to provide practical help with all rites of passage, such as baby namings, funerals (celebrations of life, non-religious funerals, spiritual ceremonies) and woodland burials.

Rastafarian

Ethiopian World Federation, 28–34 St Agnes Place, Kennington, London SE11 4BE. Tel: 0207 735 0905; www.home.clar.net/ewfinc/rasinfo.htm

Religious Society of Friends (Quakers)

Religious Society of Friends (Quakers); www.quaker.org.uk

Salvation Army

Salvation Army; www.salvationarmy.org.uk

Sikh

Network of Sikh Organisations UK, First Floor Office Suite, 192 The Broadway, Wimbledon, London SW19 1RY. Tel: 0208 540 3974.

Zoroastrian

Zoroastrian Trust Funds of Europe, Zoroastrian House, 88 Compayne Gardens, West Hampstead, London NW6 3RU. Tel: 0207 328 6018; www.ztfe.com

Index

DATE DUE
